Facelift Hotel

by
Maggie Lockridge

authorHOUSE®

AuthorHouse™
1663 Liberty Drive
Bloomington, IN 47403
www.authorhouse.com
Phone: 833-262-8899

Published by AuthorHouse 09/28/2022

ISBN: 978-1-4208-7935-3 (sc)

Print information available on the last page.

Preface

Facelift Hotel is a collection of true stories written with love and humor by Maggie Lockridge, RN. Maggie previously owned and Administered to Shanteque, Beverly Hills most luxurious cosmetic surgery recovery retreat. Maggie lived "Facelift Hotel" for eighteen years of her life. Every day that she went to work was a live performance, with the elite of this planet as the main characters, center stage. This book is not about divulging identities, it's about sharing the humor and drama of the recuperative period of cosmetic surgery.

People navigated their ways to Beverly Hills from all corners of the earth, seeking cosmetic surgery by the 'surgeons to the stars'. Many truly needed their services and others just tried to embellish what they already had. Some were trying to outrun Grandmother Nature, others were trying to outwit her with trickery via the scalpel.

It was Maggie's job to assist them through the sometimes frightening reality of recuperation. Not all are fully prepared for the path from the operating room back into society. Humor plays a major role during this journey. Some accepted the reality of their ignorance of the pain, swelling, bruising, etc. Others resented their lack of knowledge and blamed their surgeons for their lack of preparation both mentally and physically. They didn't expect the roller coaster of emotions, distorted physicality, and discomfort.

Some days she would have a reformed drug addict dealing with the Vicodin they were now required to take to fend off the pain, alcoholics hiding booze in every corner of the room, wives hiding procedures from husbands. Situations arose that no writer could possibly conjure up, they were just too incredibly unbelievable.

Attacking Grandmother Nature, the mid-section of this book, is dedicated to sharing Maggie's vast knowledge of cosmetic surgery recuperation with her readers. Maggie indicates which procedures should be addressed first when fending off the aging process. You are guided from your thirties to your sixties and beyond. She also wanted her readers to know the facts when undergoing these procedures, the amount of time involved in the healing process, the placement of suture lines, the amount of discomfort/bruising etc.

The last section of this book was compiled for anyone who has considered a cosmetic surgical procedure and is able to travel to Beverly Hills. Maggie took the knowledge of her eighteen years of caring for the Beverly Hills cosmetic surgeon's patients and compiled data on her favorite surgeons. She provides you with their education, certifications, and exactly what procedures they excel at. No where else could you obtain this information in one source. Read and laugh all the way to your plastic surgeon.

Section I

The Dramedy of Shanteque

Love...Shanteque Style

It was a beautiful Saturday in May and maybe it was the birds that were singing or the bees buzzing around the floral bushes that prompted me to introduce our only two in-house guests to one another.

Jennifer was from Chicago. She was an attorney who had told her husband that she was off to Los Angeles to a spa for two weeks. Jennifer was very attractive, in her late thirties, just the right height, the right build, the right jewelry, clothes, suitcases, shoes etc. The woman knew how to put herself together.

She decided she was going to have a facelift before Grandmother Nature made her entrance. Jennifer heard that if you attacked the aging process early enough the swelling and bruising was minimal because they didn't have to "do a lot of work". She figured by the end of two weeks the signs of recuperation would have diminished enough that make-up would do the trick and her husband would never be the wiser. Her surgery had been on the previous Wednesday and she was progressing beautifully.

Alan was in his early fifties, pleasant looking, smart, who decided to spruce up his face to keep up with the young hotties in this town. He spent his days managing real estate that his mother owned and would someday be his. He had a great sense of humor and I truly liked him for his honesty. Alan's surgery had been on Thursday and he, too, was doing well.

First I asked Jennifer if she would like to meet Alan. She said she was interested and I already knew that Alan would want to meet her. I don't think Alan would pass up meeting a lady under any circumstances. I guess he proved that because he still had his head dressing on with drains hanging from each ear.

I served each of their lunches in the day room so they could meet on neutral ground and have a parlor atmosphere instead of a bedroom environment. Little did I know that would not be a deterrent.

I was off on Sunday and returned to work the 3pm-11pm shift on Monday. Jennifer was in Alan's room, they said they had enjoyed each other's company over the weekend and would be dining together that evening. I had both of their trays delivered to Alan's room at 7:00 pm as requested. A few minutes after dinner was delivered to their door, a waiter walked past the nurse's station with a bottle of wine and two glasses on a tray. I watched him go down the hall and into Alan's room. I phoned the room and told Alan that I didn't think that wine was wise at this time. Alan assured me he had enjoyed some the evening before and was just fine. An hour later another bottle of wine is carried down the hall and into Alan's room. At this point I am concerned, but it is a hotel and we can only counsel, we cannot force an adult guest to rearrange his behavior.

Approximately forty five minutes later, around 9 pm, Jennifer came to the nurse's station door and beckoned me into the hall. She was flushed and stammered as she told me I had best go and check on Alan.

I quickly went to Alan's room and when I opened the door I stared in total disbelief. Alan was standing there holding a sheet around his naked, trembling body. He had a look of sheer panic on his face. Both ears were dripping a steady stream of blood onto the white sheet, stitches had been blown wide open.

Evidently the evening had become quite passionate, sweet love had been made, and in the heat of passion, Alan had ruptured the suture lines around both ears. An increase in blood pressure can cause this to occur. I applied a new pressure dressing to Alan's ears and told him, in a most pronounced manner, that he had probably just experienced the most expensive amour he would ever enjoy as a trip back to the operating room was currently in the making. Now that he realized his ears were still attached to his head and the situation under control, he was able to laugh at the evening's events.

A little investigating the next day brought to light that on the way back from his doctor's appointment the day before, Alan had bribed the chauffeur with a twenty dollar bill to stop at a drugstore and pick him up a box of condoms. At least they had practiced safe surgical sex.

Quite a Honeymoon

Sheila checked in with a surgical procedure of Mastopexy, breast reduction. Sheila was a major actress on TV. She had previously had her own sitcom. Prior to that she had been a member of the cast of America's number one comedy sitcom. Although she was not currently featured on television it was only a matter of time before she would be signed again for another series. She was fat, she was funny, and you didn't forget her once you saw her in a comedic role.

The staff loved her, everything had a funny connotation according to Sheila. If she was having pain it was because her preceptors were at war, if she was weak or dizzy when she got up it was because, "With all this fat how do you expect my blood to find my brain."

When you have a breast reduction the nipples are virtually removed and resutured in a higher position. It is very important that a new blood supply be established to this transplanted nipple. Sheila was on her way to recovery and left Aftercare after three days.

Because of her weight, an additional amount of concern is involved due to compromised circulation. She left the facility with pink, healthy, transplanted nipples and healing suture lines.

Sheila was excited because she was getting married in a few weeks. She spoke positively and negatively about the relationship. She said it wasn't ideal but at her age you made concessions. He was younger than she was and that flattered her. In fact, it revitalized her.

Three weeks later we received a call from her surgeon informing us that Sheila would be coming back. She had an infection in one of her nipples and she refused to go to a general hospital. One of her nipples had separated from her breast. Sheila knew that if she went to a hospital her problem would leak to the press. I reluctantly took her back, but not before I had a conversation with her celebrity surgeon. I was not set up to take in guests with an infection. He assured me he had her on a strong antibiotic that would negate any live bacteria. I encased her mattress in plastic, set up as many nursing precautions that I could, and picked her up from her surgeon's appointment.

Sheila soon confided in me that she had been married and was on her honeymoon when some unforeseen activity had somehow dislodged her nipple from her breast. She had a sense of humor about it, it didn't take much imagination to figure out how this one happened. For the next ten days a nurse from the surgeon's office showed up twice a day to irrigate the wound, redress it, and offer emotional support to Sheila.

Sheila left the facility on her road to recovery. I read three months later that a divorce had taken place.

Al Qaeda

He first became a guest of Shanteque's in Feb. of 04. He had a rhinoplasty (nose surgery), kept to himself, refused pain medication, and checked out after two days. There were no red flags at that time. His physicality looked Mideastern, he came to us from Ontario, Canada, and paid cash. Many of my guests pay cash, they don't want a paper trail. He was a very handsome man, deep set eyes, dark tanned skin, thick black hair, masculine features, a toned body and great hands. I always notice a man's hands first. My mother always said, "If they don't take care of their hands just imagine what their feet look like."

However, in April of 04 he returned. This time his procedures included raising his forehead, cheek implants, a nasal revision and facial liposuction etc., serious image changing procedures. Now I was curious. He was 34 years old and a very good looking Mideastern appearing man to begin with. Why would anyone do something like this at his age. The wheels began to turn. He told one of my nurses that he was Italian. Every time I entered the room you could see his legs jump as if he was nervous or apprehensive. He kept to himself, no visitors, no phone calls, came in through Ontario and paid cash once again. I had my suite attendant bring me his glass when she changed his water, I wanted his fingerprints.

My thoughts indicated, "He's changing his image so he can slip in and out of the country as an Italian. He doesn't have his heavy set forehead anymore, his nose is non-Mideastern (straighter), his face will be completely different in depth, individual features, and size." I'm calling Homeland Security. In the back of my mind I have always wondered if history would have been different if the flying school operative had been a little more alert, astute, imaginative, patriotic, curious or caring about the 9/11 Arabs who came to him for flying lessons. The ones who didn't want to learn how to land the plane, only fly it.

I called information for Washington DC and asked for Homeland Security, I asked the person who answered to connect me to an individual in charge of investigating suspicious individuals. I was transferred to Mr. Ryan's voicemail. I left a brief but concise message regarding my suspicions and gave him my phone number. Not more than 30 minutes later I received a call from Mr. Ryan.

I gave him a detailed accounting of my suspicions of this man. He seemed interested in the information. I then asked him if he would like the surgeon's name who performed the surgery. He said it wouldn't be necessary. I then informed him that the surgeon would have "before" and "after" photos of this man. He then took the name. I informed him I had a glass with fingerprints on it and was told he didn't need it, it wasn't necessary for the investigation.

I was disappointed at his lackluster interest in my "terrorist". I was even more upset at the surgeon who had performed the surgery, most likely accepting a large amount of cash to perform it, and, to my knowledge, never informed anyone of his own suspicions, he must have had them.

A few days later I phoned Mr. Ryan again as I had forgotten to give him the patient's credit card number. I asked him if they had turned up anything suspicious. He informed me that he couldn't divulge any information, positive or negative. Case closed.

Veronica

Veronica behaved normally when first admitted. She was under the influence of anesthesia, pain medication, and other medications administered during her surgery. Her behavior did not set off any bells or whistles the first 18 hours she was with us. She had undergone extensive surgery and was in the deep throws of recovery. However, as soon as the heavy duty medications wore off and the REAL Veronica came through, we knew we were in for a rough ride.

Her behavior was erratic and her mood swings unpredictable. There was no rhyme or reason for her behavior based on the medications we were administering. She was high, she was low, she was assertive, she was passive, she was profane, she was sweet. No one could figure out just what was going on.

Was she self medicating? When Veronica was at her doctor's appointment the second post-operative day I decided to search the patient's suitcases. No medications were found. However, Veronica was always clutching her purse and would not let it out of her grasp, sleeping with it beside her on the bed. Not a good sign.

I phoned her doctor and spoke with his nurse. I asked her if she had suspected any irregularities in Veronica's personality before surgery. She said, "Yes, There were several issues over payment of the surgeon's bill, the patient became very defensive when told that her surgeries would actually cost money." The doctor had considered refusing her as a patient but on the second visit she was a different person and all had progressed normally after that.

I told the nurse of Veronica's erratic, weird, unpredictable behavior and she decided to phone Veronica's husband and see if there was anything in her past that had not been divulged. Her husband stated that she had been a drug abuser but he didn't think she was on anything at this time. They had five little children at home and he did not feel that Veronica would get back on drugs with the children to care for.

The following day Veronica felt much better and decided to go shopping. She came back with hundreds of dollars worth of clothes, pajamas, lounging outfits, sportswear etc. She still kept her purse under her arm and I was determined to discover whether she was taking medications we were not aware of. I was ultimately responsible for this woman's well being and I wanted to know my enemies. I found the opportunity the next day when Veronica was in the bathtub. She had forgotten her purse on her bed and I seized the opportunity. Her purse contained several different types of narcotics from two different medical doctors from the Los Angeles area. Both were dated during her stay at Shanteque. I had never heard of the doctors indicated on the labels. Why would they prescribe narcotics of this nature on the first visit. What story had she told them? One thing was certain, her shopping sprees included a little bit more than just department stores.

Her behavior became more erratic that afternoon and I called the doctor telling him that Shanteque could not be responsible for this woman's well being. She was taking unlimited amounts of narcotics, hiding the fact, and leaving the facility at will. I felt someone had to come and sit with her or a serious situation could result. The doctor called Veronica's husband and informed him he had to come to his wife's assistance.

The husband was at first angry, "What had the doctor prescribed that had made his wife this way?" He was informed that the doctor hadn't prescribed anything past her initial post-operative pain medication which had been long used up. That this was not a surgery related situation. It involved a predisposing condition that the surgeon was not made aware of. The husband reluctantly hopped on a red eye and was at Shanteque the next afternoon.

Veronica's husband was not what I expected. He was charming, quiet, kind eyes, the kind of teddy bear type. I had pictured someone a little more rustic, controlling. He joined Veronica for the night. It was quiet in the room at first, then loud voices were heard, very serious discussions were being had. The next morning her husband tried to wake Veronica but she was still sound, sound asleep, snoring loudly. He showered and told the nurses he was going down for breakfast. The nurses entered her room to try to awaken her for breakfast. She told them on no uncertain terms to allow her to sleep. The room was a tornado. Every edible from the honor bar was strewn about the room, pretzels, potato chips, M&M's, etc. You literally had to pick your footing across the floor. Every article of clothing she had brought with her and had purchased subsequently, was also strewn about the floor and furniture. It must have been quite a melee.

Veronica woke up enough to get herself out of bed around 10:00 am. She showered and dressed. Her husband returned and they checked out of Shanteque and into the main hotel. When he came back for more of her belongings I was able to discuss her condition with him. I also recommended that he call her surgeon. He had taken Veronica's pills out of her purse so she was totally without medication. I told him I felt she needed professional help. I felt so sorry for him. What a huge problem he had on his hands and such responsibility. A drug abusing wife and five little ones at home to worry about.

The following morning the hotel maid informed me that the police had to be called the night before and Veronica had been taken away in handcuffs. It seems she became violent when no further drugs were available and had attacked her husband. I learned later from her surgeon that she had gone to a drug rehabilitation facility and then returned to her family.

Her Highness the Bitchess

There is always that guest who you cannot please no matter who tries or how hard they try. This particular guest started in the limo on the way to Shanteque: The driver was driving too fast, didn't she know that her passenger had just had surgery. Why wasn't there any water in the car for her? How could the recovery room discharge her in such pain, no one there seemed to know what the *** they were doing, did we have her bags and where was her purse. She had her jewelry in her purse and it had better all still be there when she reached her room.

When they arrived at Shanteque and tried to help her out of the car it was more of the same. Don't touch her, she'll do it herself, the least they could do was lift her feet up onto the wheelchair foot holder, put the blanket on her she was cold, give her the *** purse she wanted to hold it, be careful with the large bag it held her computer, don't go too fast she was dizzy. It never stopped.

When wheeled into her room her comments started once again. Turn off that *** music, I want quiet. Take the roses out of the room she has allergies, blow out the candle she can't tolerate smells. Get her black pajamas out of the suitcase, they're underneath the clothes that she wants hung in the closet. Get that pitcher of ice water out of here, I only drink bottled water and NO ICE.

When assisted into bed and made comfortable with pillows under her knees, her head, and both arms for support, she admitted she was comfortable. However, that was brief, a few minutes later she is on the nurse call button, she needs someone to pour more water for her, turn on the television, pull the drapes it's too *** bright, dial the phone for her she can't see to dial, where were the pills she takes everyday, she wants them where she can reach them on the nightstand, did anyone think to plug in her cell phone did we think it ran on * * * air. Her charger was in her suitcase, why hadn't someone unpacked it? It was endless.

The nurses did their best but no matter what they did for her it wasn't done right or well. The towels weren't soft enough, she didn't like the smell of the soap, they rubbed too hard or too soft. The tub water was too deep or not deep enough, too warm or not warm enough. Her mouth was foul and she made several comments to the effect that her friends had been to other facilities and perhaps she had made the wrong choice.

The nurse's station is a place for the nurses to vent. When in the guest's rooms they are in a service oriented mode and must suppress all inner feelings. However, they can let them come forth in the nurse's station. Since Her Bitchess had arrived, the nurse's station had never heard such an orchestration. I should have made a recording of the comments that were made by her assigned nurses. They said all the things that they held back when in Her Bitchess's presence. Finally, late in the afternoon of the second day her assigned nurse came to me and said, "You don't pay me enough to take this kind of verbal abuse." I knew then that I had to fall back on my old technique that worked every time.

I went to Her Bitchess's room and said, "Her Bitch", (no not really) "It seems that Shanteque is not able to meet your needs. Since this is a time of recuperation and your comfort and happiness are extremely important toward a successful recovery, would you like me to make arrangements for you to be transferred to another facility? Your peace of mind is my priority."

No one has ever wanted me to arrange a transfer. Once we have, most tactfully, let them know that their behavior is not acceptable and we would like them to go elsewhere, they turn the corner and become human beings again. I also informed her that my staff was not used to profane language and were finding it offensive. By law, I had to do whatever I could to give my staff an acceptable work environment.

Her Bitchess did not want to go anywhere else and she actually mellowed out. Some people are so used to being in total control at all times that when they discover they are not in control, such as after surgery, defense mechanisms set in and alternative behavior patterns take over. By the time she went home two days later, she was singing the nurse's praise and thanking me for getting her through a very difficult time.

Sweet William

William booked himself the largest suite we had to offer. He decided, after being jilted by his gay lover, that it was time for a facelift and several other body enhancement procedures.

He was a gentle, sweet, thoughtful guest with a wonderful sense of humor. His surgery went well and after two days of recuperation he was up and about his room, starting to take walks in the hallway, and chatting with the nurses in the nurse's station.

William said that the primary reason for his surgery was because his lover had literally thrown him out without notice. The lover was known by all in La La Land due to his musical notoriety. Gentle William told stories of how, after the break up, he had gone down to his lover's beach house and moved all of the furniture out on the sand, said he didn't break anything, just wanted to cause a little bedlam. He hoped that the surgery would boost his morale and help him make new friends.

William insisted on ordering dinner for the nurses at night. He had the nurses call whatever restaurant they wanted and have them deliver their favorite entree. He told them to use the credit card on file. On his 5th day he went out for a walk and came back with certificates for facials for everyone from the Aida Thibiant salon, one of Beverly Hills most chic. He continued to make shopping side trips and brought back bags and boxes of new clothes. All the latest in fashion, he definitely seemed to be getting back into the mainstream of life.

He extended his stay and was with us for more than a week. He didn't want to go home until he was totally presentable. He promised everyone he would stop by in a few weeks when totally healed. He called the staff "his angels". The day William left he signed a credit card receipt for more than $5000.00. Since only the number of the credit card and the expiration date appeared on the reservation form, no one suspected fraud.

However, within two weeks the facility received a telephone call from the lover. He was furious, said he had not authorized any of the charges that William had made and he would not honor them. It was evident that William had retained his lover's credit card and started life anew at his ex lover's expense.

I often wondered if they had ever confronted each other again. Seeing a facelift that you had just paid for on an ex-lover's face must be a bit annoying. It could have been worse, he could have gotten a penile enhancement.

National League Story

The recovery room phoned at 8 pm to inform us that our guest had entered the recovery room, her surgery was finished and successful, and requesting a pick-up time for our guest of 9 pm. This was later than usual but not unusual for this particular surgeon. He often operated late into the night.

Upon arriving at the surgeon's office my chauffeur and nurse were informed by the recovery room nurse that two family members would be following us to the hotel in their car and please drive accordingly not to lose them. The guest was a middle aged woman who had undergone body surgery. She was still very groggy and fell asleep whenever given the opportunity. She had to be assisted by two nurses into the wheelchair and then into the Shanteque limo.

Upon entering the underground private hotel parking lot and assisting the guest into a wheelchair they were met by the two family members at the elevator, each was toting their own luggage. The chauffeur requested that they take the next elevator as they would be quite crowded if all entered at one time. The family said they would not wait and pushed onto the elevator with the nurse, the guest in a wheelchair, their luggage, and the chauffeur. It was all downhill from there. Murphy's law took over.

Nine times out of ten the elevator will go directly to the second floor, but as luck would have it, it stopped in the lobby. A man was standing there waiting for an elevator. The chauffeur requested that he wait for the next elevator but before he could finish the request the man had pushed his way in. As he pushed his way in on one side of the elevator he brushed against the catheter bag hanging on the wheelchair causing it to fall on the floor. The wheelchair also rolled slightly backwards toward the doors of the elevator. As the chauffeur bent over to pick up the catheter bag and hang it back on the side of the wheelchair, his finger came off the "hold door open" button and the doors began to shut on the handle bars of the wheelchair. The chauffeur then disengaged the handle bars and the elevator continued on its way to the second floor. At this point the family is livid, calling the staff names, furious with the stranger on the elevator, making a scene for everyone to hear. The profanity was profuse. Bear in mind that the guest is totally oblivious to all of this, she is enjoying a twilight sleep and the next day did not even remember the trip to the retreat.

When the guest was rolled into her room her assigned nurse was waiting to assist her into bed. Because the woman was so groggy the nurse reached under the guest's arms to help her out of the wheelchair. The family started screaming that the nurse was going to ruin the guest's surgery because she had undergone an "arm tightening". The guest had also undergone a tummy tuck and there was just no way she was going to get into bed completely on her own. The charge nurse then entered the room and between both nurses the guest was made comfortable, positioned, and assessed. This was done, however, with both family members continuing to yell at the charge nurse, using more creative profanity, and enlightening her on the series of events in the elevator.

The following morning my assistant entered the guest's room to obtain a signature on the registration card, a routine matter. The family member was there and informed her in her usual haughty, condescending manner, that no one was going to sign anything after the treatment the guest had received the night before. My assistant had been versed on the events of the prior evening so no questions were needed on her part. She informed the family member that if the card was not signed she would have to remove the guest from the premises as soon as possible. That this was a hotel and no hotel that she knew of allowed a guest to remain in house without a signature on file. The family member then signed the form.

The guest remained in the retreat for three days. She received the finest of care, was delighted with everyone, and informed her assigned nurse that she was having additional surgery in six months and would be back. Meanwhile, whenever the family members arrived and behaved so rudely toward the staff, she would never say a word in the staff's defense. They continued to use foul language to everyone, even on phone calls they made to others, profanity came so naturally to them. It was their way of communicating. Several times staff left the room because of the family's total lack of appreciation of care for their relative, or respect for any of the staff. They did not desire to be in the presence of such language.

Finally check out day arrived. My assistant once again entered the guest's room to present the bill to the family member who had arrived to take our guest home. The family member refused to sign the bill and asked where the discount was. Since my assistant knew nothing about a discount she said she would have to consult with the Administrator. She was visibly upset when she came into my office and told me that they had refused to sign the bill. She was personally so fed up with the behavior of the family that she said she did not want to go back into the room and would I please handle it.

I walked into the room with the bill in hand and asked why they were refusing to sign for it. The family member said, "Havn't you talked with our attorney?" I said, "No, why should I have?" She then haughtily pulled out her cell phone and dialed her attorney's number. As soon as she had him on line she handed me the phone. I took it, introduced myself, and told him I wasn't quite sure why we were having this discussion. The attorney said that the family fully expected to receive a complimentary night for the first night the guest had been with us. That I was lucky I did not have a law suit slapped against me for negligence, practice to endanger, damages sustained by the guest etc. etc., I was speechless. He said that in order to defer legal action being taken by the family I had best deduct the rate of the first night's reservation. I must admit it took a great deal of inner composure to maintain my ladylike qualities. I quietly hung up the phone, returned it, and left the room. I had my assistant credit the account for the first night's rate. One thing I knew, this ball player had millions to my hundreds if it came to fighting a lawsuit, especially one without merit and as frivolous as this one. There had certainly been no damages to my guest. I often think you can always tell when it's "new money.. no class."

When my assistant had adjusted the bill, I took it back into the room and handed it to the family member. The guest was sitting on the couch approximately 12 to 15 feet across the room, in fact there was a table between us. The family member signed the credit slip. I then said to the family member, "The guest has indicated to her nurse that she is planning additional surgery in six months and would like to return, however, I'm sure she will be happier recuperating elsewhere." I then left the room. I would not subject my staff to such behavior again.

I returned to my office and my other duties. Five minutes later I saw my assistant start to get up from her desk with a startled look on her face. A split second later the family member literally charged into my office and thrust her cell phone in my face. She said, "Someone wants to talk to you." I took the phone and said, "Hello". A very distinctive voice on the other end said, "Do you know who this is?" I said, "Yes, I believe it's _ _ _ _." He said, "Your right, **how dare you shake your finger in my "guests" face.** What kind of a facility are you running. You sound totally incompetent to be running a business. You're lucky you're not facing a lawsuit." His voice was threatening, loud, rude, frighteningly out of control. He rambled on with his comments for at least a minute and a half. In the meantime, the family member is standing on the other side of my desk with her arms folded across her chest and the most smug look on her face. The look said, "I'll get the final say here".

As soon as the ball player said, "How dare you shake your finger in the 'guest's' face," I knew what I was dealing with. The family member had distorted, reinvented, misrepresented, and lied about the events that had occurred. To my knowledge this particular ball player had never visited this family member while she had been a guest, had no idea what Shanteque was all about, had never met one of the guest's nurses, had never spoken to or met me, or obtained a sense about the essence of Shanteque. Since all incoming calls are screened and no one had taken his call, we did not feel he had even spoken to the guest to see whether or not she had been happy with her stay.

I allowed the ball player to finish with his comments. I then said, "Sir, I'm sorry that you feel this way. Your relative is on her way out now, I will see to it that she is safely in the car." I then closed the cell phone and went to hand the phone back to it's owner. My assistant was standing at my side by this time, she was seriously concerned about my safety in the presence of this individual. As I raised my arm with the phone to return it, the family member raised her right hand and grabbed the phone so hard out of my hand that my swivel chair swung around and I found myself facing the wall. The family member then exited quickly. My assistant was furious, she wanted me to sue her for assault. I was just so happy to be done with the lot of them.

It was only a few months later that this particular ball player was charged with a serious crime. I have to admit that at the moment I believed in divine justice.

I thought that that was the end of the ball player saga. However, about three months later I am once again at my desk when I hear male voices in the nurse's station and look up from my desk. My assistant has another one of those "Holy Cow" expressions on her face and my curiosity peeked. She rose and entered my office. She said, "There are two men from the FBI here to talk to you. I had absolutely no idea what this was all about. The ball player saga had been totally dismissed from my frame of reference. When I went out to meet them they introduced themselves, showed me their badges and asked me if there was someplace where we could talk privately. They were stiff as a board and stern of face, about as official appearing as they could make themselves. I showed them to one of my empty rooms. Once in the room they asked me to close and lock the door. By now my knees are knocking, I can't remember either of their names, and I'm trying to think back through all the events of my life to figure out why they could be here.

Once the door was locked and I turned around, the agents softened a little, actually smiled, and informed me that word had gotten to them about an incident I had with this particular ball player. I was so relieved by that time that I had to laugh. I asked them how they had ever learned about the incident. They would not tell me their source but wanted to ask me questions about the call.

I told them the entire story using actual names and relationships and both men could not help but chuckle, really hard, about the elevator scene. I then described the ball player's conversation, his tone of voice etc. They asked me if he had used foul language or threatened me personally. I said no, he hadn't. He was just plain rude, misinformed, and juvenile. I felt he had been the victim of this particular family member's lies.

The agents then gave me their cards and left.

Porno Princess

I walked into Blossom's room to hear her on the phone saying, "Of course I did it honey, just wait until you see them. I named them Twist and Shout cause that's what it's all about right honey. Uh huh, my only problem is I can't get out of bed, they are sooo heavy and weigh sooo much, I guess I'm just going to have to rest one on each of your big broad shoulders huh sweetie. Did you tell Big Feller and Killer Buns I'm doing this? Boy, I can't wait to see their faces when the camera starts to roll and Twist and Shout get a chance to perform."

I knew right then that this was a live one. If I didn't have a smile on my face when I entered the room, I was grinning from ear to ear now. I was carrying her breakfast tray and set it on the table. I wanted her to eat at the table because she should be up and about, getting exercise to prevent blood clots, restore good circulation, and get her strength back. Her surgery had been the day before.

Blossom had her old breast implants removed and larger ones inserted. I saw the two implants that had been removed sitting in a plastic bag on the end table. I asked Blossom if she had any special plans for those. She informed me that they would be used as conversation pieces on her coffee table, and if any of her dates came early or she wasn't ready yet, well, then they could get started without her. The most outrageously funny part about it was she truly was not kidding. Blossom was one of those free spirits who could say anything, and no matter how off-the-wall it was, it was cute because she said it. She was blonde, naturally, not naturally blond, but naturally. She was about 5'4", petit, big blue eyes that were always dancing about the room until they found their next topic of conversation. Then they would look back at you and stare you right in the eye until her point had been made. Then off about the room they went until the next thought popped into her head.

I went to help her as she was struggling to upright herself. The size of her new implants weighed 4 lbs. each. Between the pain and the eight pounds on her chest she was having a rough time sitting up. I showed her how to use the electric bed to help her get upright. Then, with a little help from me, she swung her legs over the side of the bed and sat there getting her breath. She took one breast in each hand to support them and walked over to the table. What a sight. I tightened the elastic bandage that she had wrapped around her breasts in hopes of giving her more support. When she was seated at the table she asked me to bring the phone closer to her as she was expecting a call from her "sweetcums". I am quietly hysterical, I cannot leave this room, she is too entertaining. I just couldn't ask her about that name. She then volunteered that she had been dating sweetcums for two years and he was the distributor of her films. She said she made "love movies" and had met him on a film set. She then went on to tell me how he probably wouldn't be able to come to see her because he had two broken legs. At this point I knew I had to go home that night and write everything down.

I asked her what had happened to her honey's legs. She said, "It's kind of a weird story, you see he makes wonderful videos and I'm the star. I mean I'm not his only star, he has Red Hot, that's because she has flaming red hair, and she's good, but not as good as me. Then there's Sugar Lips, and Golden Goddess and Slippery Syl. That's because she only does it on a waterbed coated with Mazola oil. Anyway, these videos are really great and Sammy, that's my boyfriend, wanted to broaden his distribution base, so he went a little out of his territory, you know... now, the guys who worked that territory learned Sammy had been there selling our videos so they broke both his legs. He's healing up just fine though cause he's got Nick to push his wheelchair around. Nick's a real cute young guy that showed up for a roll in a movie and Sam gave him the job of pushing him around. Guess Nick thinks he's earning his movie roll, sort of like a woman when she gets on a casting couch, you know."

Two evenings later I looked down the hall to see a man in a wheelchair being pushed by a younger man into Blossom's room. I thought it nice that he was coming to see her. About thirty minutes later I received a call from security, asking me to curtail the activities on the balcony of room 608. It seems guests in the pool and cabanas below, were having too much fun. I knew that was Blossom's room so I went to 608, knocked on the door, and was told by a man to come in. When I entered, Blossom was no where to be seen, and neither was the young man that had navigated the wheelchair. Sam was watching TV and did not seem concerned. I made my way to the balcony to find young Nick and my cute little Blossom making whoopee in the corner. I told Blossom that security had called and whoopee on the balcony was frowned upon at this particular hotel. I had to make light of it as I did not want a full blown scene if Sam should find out what was happening out there. It was dark outside and the curtain was drawn halfway closed against the double glass sliding door so he could not see them. Nothing more was ever mentioned about the episode. Blossom left the next morning.

Wino

Laura was admitted to Shanteque on a pre-op basis. Guests sometimes elect to check in the night before their surgery so they can unpack their belongings, become adjusted to the room, relax, and have a delicious dinner. They are comfortable with the fact that the nurses will wake them at the appointed hour and provide transportation to their surgery. Her "significant other" was with her and spent the night. They seemed to have a caring relationship.

Laura impressed me, she was the owner of a large company that specialized in city and county contracts. There was no doubt that this woman dealt with millions on a daily basis. I soon found out that there was also no doubt that the "significant other" was also a recipient of her success.

Laura went to surgery without incident and returned later that day. Up to this point I had no suspicions. During the evening I was informed that she must be a "light weight" with medication because they had only given her one Vicodin but she was slightly hallucinatory. She would respond appropriately if questioned and her vital signs were within normal but in between times she would be talking to herself and picking things out of the air.

The following morning, as I was making my rounds, I entered Laura's room to find her frantically calling her bank to place a hold on all of her accounts. She was distraught, crying, and muttering some serious profanity directed to her boyfriend. She told me that she had put $40,000.00 in her boyfriend's account the week before and he had already spent it and wanted more. He had been at her bank trying to get money transferred to his account which infuriated her under the circumstances of her current infirmity. She wanted to restrict three different accounts that he had access to. I thought she was justified and allowed her to continue with her calls. However, she did seem a bit "off".

Laura had a doctor's appointment later that morning so I decided to research the situation a little further. I went to her room and looked around. At first nothing seemed inappropriate, but my eye caught something that glistened from the bottom of the curtain. When I drew back the drape, there were three wine bottles sitting side by side, one empty, one half empty, and one not yet opened. I then looked around the room, found another unopened bottle behind her bed, and two more in a bag in the closet. This woman had come prepared. I gathered all of the bottles and brought them to my office. I then hoped no one would enter and see my stash. When Laura came back from the doctor's office I went in and explained to her that I had found her wine, and that it was being held for her when she left. Laura was most compliant. I also explained that we could not risk the combination of pain medication and alcohol being taken at the same time, resulting in possible serious complications. She was just a little too compliant. All went well the rest of the day.

The following morning I happened to see Laura walking past the office door, I could hardly keep a straight face. She had dressed herself in jeans and a blouse. However, she had also taken another pair of white jeans, and with the waist band resting on her shoulders, she had wrapped the two legs around her head in a turban style. She still had a full head dressing on with two bulbous drains dangling on each side, peeking out between the legs of the jeans. I asked her where she was headed, she said the room was closing in on her and she needed to take a little walk. Since we are a hotel I could not stop her. However, when she disappeared in the elevator I asked my transportation engineer, (driver), to please follow her and make sure she did not go to the bar in the lobby. The driver returned a few minutes later and informed me she had left the hotel, hailed a cab and driven off. This was a first for me. I felt extremely responsible for her well-being. I decided to call the number on her reservation card and at least inform a member of her family that she had left the facility. I dialed the number and was a little speechless when Laura answered the phone, it was her cell number. I asked her where she was going and that I was concerned about her well being. She told me she was just fine. She was going to Santa Monica but would return within an hour and not to worry. My concern was that she was going either to her boyfriend's to confront him, or to a liquor store for more wine. Her boyfriend had not been in to see her for two days.

An hour later, Laura returned. I fully expected her to be carrying a shopping bag full of wine bottles, but she had nothing, so my curiosity peaked. The jeans were still around her head. What the general public must have thought about her appearance was beyond my comprehension. Somebody must have had a good laugh. I was only happy I hadn't received a call from a local precinct requesting me to come and get her.

What I wasn't aware of was that Laura had handed over her shopping bag full of wine to a bellman in the lobby, requesting that he deliver it directly to her room in thirty minutes, and tipped him appropriately. Laura was a smart lady. She had a very pleasant, rose-embellished, evening.

The following morning Laura went home, I returned her wine to her and at that point discovered her new stash. As long as she was doing just fine and departing from Shanteque, I had no further obligation, I had already counseled her. She was an adult and could now do as she wished. She gave us all hugs and departed with her driver. Her surgeon knew of the wine intake.

Two weeks later this beautiful woman appeared in the nurse's station with her "significant other" on her arm. She brought gifts for the girls and if we hadn't recognized the boyfriend we would not have known the identity of this lovely lady. She appeared in complete control of all her faculties, perfectly coifed and attired, and very grateful to Shanteque for being there in her time of need. Laura was just fine.

But Doctor, One Nostril is
Higher Than the Other

When, my driver is busy on an appointment, and there is a conflicting appointment on the board, I jump into my "chauffeur cap" and take the second patient to their surgeon's office. I delivered my guest safely into the treatment room at the surgeon's office and took a seat in the waiting room.

A few minutes later a young man, perhaps 17-19 years old, took a seat across from me. He was accompanied by his mother, who chose to stand at his side, versus take a chair three feet away, also across from him. Mother was dressed in tight fitting, three quarter floral print capri pants, clear vinyl backless heeled shoes, large diamond stud earrings, a loose fitting rhinestone studded t-shirt and carrying a Gucci bag. It was evident to me that the young man had undergone a rhinoplasty the day before. His eyes and nose bridge were swollen and bruised. He looked miserable, having to dab at his nose constantly for drainage and talking in a very nasal quality voice.

The doctor started to walk past to enter one of the treatment rooms when the mother stepped in his path. The ensuing conversation went like this:

Mother: "Doctor, can you take a quick look at Jeff's nose, is this amount of swelling normal?"

Doctor: "Yes, he's really not badly swollen at all with the extent of his surgery."

Mother: "But doctor, look at his eyes, I can't believe that they would bruise like that, we never thought that it would be so disfiguring."

Doctor: "If you remember we had to do a lot of cartilage work, that always causes more bruising than if it's just soft tissue."

Mother.   "But look at his nostrils doctor, one is higher than the other"

Doctor: "Yes, it is slightly at this time but it will reappoint itself when the swelling goes down."

Mother: "Doctor, the tip of his nose points up, it's not going to stay there is it? His father's used to point up a little and he had to have it fixed, we don't want Jeff's nose to be like that."

Doctor;   "No, it won't be pointing up. It will be just fine, the tape that is on the bridge of his nose is perhaps holding it slightly upward due to the swelling."

Jeff: "Mother, I'm sure everything will be just fine, thank you doctor."

Mother: "I'm still worried about that nostril, are you positive they will be even? You can see that one is definitely higher, right doctor? What would make it do that, I can't understand how one side of the nose could be lifted like that, I certainly hope that this isn't going to require another surgery."

At this point the doctor is getting a little impatient, I'm hysterical behind my magazine and he can see my eyes are laughing over the top of it. He is trying to keep a straight face.

Doctor: "Don't worry, please, you can't tell anything about results for at least ten days. The swelling has to diminish to allow the tissues to take their new position. Jeff will have a great new nose by the end of next week."

Mother: "How long should we keep icing his eyes?"

Doctor: You can ice for about a week, it will feel good and help with the swelling."

Mother: "About how much ice should there be in the bag, I don't want it too heavy on his nose."

Doctor: Fill the icemask about half full."

Mother: Would that be about two icecubes in each eye pocket, it's really hard to tell because you can't see inside the mask."

Doctor: "It's easier if you use chopped ice, it's lighter on the eyes."

Jeff: "Thank you doctor, I know what you mean."

During this time you can see Jeff getting more and more agitated at his mother's incessant questions. It is clearly evident we have an overly possessive, anally controlling mother of a well rounded son who is trying desperately to be respectful of both the doctor and his mother.

There was no doubt in my mind as to who wore the capri's in that family.

One Rocky Rock Star

The first time this female stayed with me I vowed I would never submit myself or my staff to that kind of abuse again. Her name was added to my VUP list. It's a list with 8-10 names on it of previous guests who were not welcome to stay with me in the future, sort of a cosmetic surgery black list. VUP stood for Very Unimportant People.

The problem was, her doctor called me personally to make the second reservation. He pleaded with me to accept her, he knew what we were up against with her as a guest. He did not want her going home because he knew that she would not give herself the appropriate treatments for laser healing, full face laser that is. She was abusive to his office staff too. How do you turn down such a direct request. I relented and knew how sorry I would be, I felt like a traitor to my staff.

This particular musician/guest was unscrupled in her personal life and certainly in her public life. It was all for one, and the one was herself. She was rude, abusive, physically assertive, a known drug and alcohol addict, arrested numerous times etc etc etc. I almost had a nurse quit because of her behavior the last time she had been a guest of Shanteque. I didn't tell my staff of the reservation, I wanted them to be happy as long as possible.

Full face laser is a tough procedure for a perfectly normal person, but for someone who is drug abusive and known for a rough/tough personna, it's not only difficult for them but for everyone around them.

I assigned her a room at the end of the hall because I wanted her as far away from my other guests as possible. It was a very pretty room with double doors leading to a balcony and fronting a neighborhood street. We were located in a small boutique hotel in a neighborhood at the time.

The first few hours of her admission went just fine, she still had anesthesia on board. As soon as it had worn off she began screaming about the pain, demanding her medication, (Demerol), yelling at people on her phone, complaining of the food, calling for a nurse and then locking her door, using the most profane language these ears had ever heard, and smoking when she knew this was a no-smoking facility.

I had twinges of sympathy for her, brief, as they passed quickly. Reality just wasn't there for her, she had no concept of time. Everything she said was a distortion of the fact, the time it took to get her pain pills, the time it took for a nurse to answer her call button. Nothing was done right or well.

I went to her room one day when her nurse told me she was smoking in the room instead of on the balcony as we had requested. When I very nicely requested that she smoke on the balcony she started swearing at me, picked up the ashtray, and sent it sailing through the double doors, over the balcony, and crashing to the street below. I was just happy the doors had been open and she hadn't hit anyone on the street.

The next evening she told the night nurse at midnight that she wanted a massage and she wanted it then. The nurse was able to coerce a masseuse on our list to come in at that hour to administer it. When she arrived at 1:00 a.m. to give our guest her massage, the guest had locked her door, and yelled out, "Who in hell wants a massage at 1:00 a.m. in the morning." She refused to allow the masseuse into her room. The masseuse had a look of profound relief on her face and left. The guest was charged the $150.00 fee for the massage.

I remember her personal assistant coming into the nurse's station with bags of personal items she had requested from home. He vented a little with us in regards to her abusive behavior. He apologized for the way she had been treating the staff as he had witnessed it at times. He said that she did have a nice side to her, it just wasn't allowed out that often. She was the first guest to have her name listed on my VUP list a second time.

Shock Therapy

Natalie arrived at 11:00 p.m. after 12 hours of surgery. The surgery included an endoscopic forehead, facelift, and bilateral upper and lower eyelid surgery. Her post-operative order sheet did not indicate how long she had been in the recovery room prior to being discharged to our care. Twelve hours of anesthesia, along with the other medications given for blood pressure, etc. can leave you pretty disorientated when you wake up. As soon as you do start waking up you are medicated for the discomfort you are complaining of. Thus you now have narcotics on board.

The following notations were made by the charge Registered Nurse upon the patient's admission: Patient highly agitated, delusional and combative. States, "Don't touch me, take these metal objects off my head, why are you putting these metal magnets on my head? There are magnets in my neckroll, people are talking to me from these magnets." The nurse's notes continued, "patient refusing to take any medications for pain or restlessness. Patient unable to stop talking or moving around. Dr. X called, three way conversation held with anesthetist, doctor and myself. Dr. ordered Phenergan 12.5 mg. IM. Administrator notified of combatant guest. Ordered private duty nurse to remain with guest. Dr. states patient being treated for brain tumor."

When my charge nurse learned of the guest's Meningioma of the brain, even though it was indicated as asymptomatic at this time, the picture took on a whole new twist. Why would someone operate on a woman for twelve hours who is being treated for a brain tumor. Her history also included mitral valve prolapse, hypertension, and a history of thrombophletitis. It took four doses of Phenergan at half hour intervals to calm this patient down so that she could rest. She rested only for short intervals and woke up in between, still disoriented and restless but not combative. She was discharged to her doctor's appointment the next morning. Only a one night reservation had been made.

Four days later I received a call from Dr. X. He asked me what went on with our treatment of his patient. He stated she came into her appointment with a metal object and told him we had attached it to her head and given her shock treatment with it. I could not believe what the doctor was saying. How could he possibly be giving any credibility to what this particular patient was saying under the circumstances of her medical condition, and the events of the night she spent at Shanteque. He actually seemed to believe that we had been guilty of mistreating his patient. I asked to see the object, but it was never sent to Shanteque, and I did not get an opportunity to get to his office to see it. Obviously it did not exist and perhaps the phone call had been made in her presence to assuage her.

Sly Made Her Day

We had a guest at Shanteque who was married to the son of one of the Mideast's wealthiest men, he was notoriously wealthy in the 80's with multiple wives, divorces, etc. It seemed that the wealthy father in law did not approve of his son's marriage to this American woman. Her name was BJ and the father in law did not support or extend his fortune to his son because of this marriage. The young couple were having a very difficult time according to BJ. However, it did not stop her from coming back from a Beverly Hills shopping spree with six pairs of designer shoes. I wasn't quite sure just what her definition of "borderline poverty" was. The sales slip was for $2500.00.

BJ enjoyed having cosmetic surgical procedures and had stayed with me several times. She was a friend of Sly Stallones before she was married and everytime BJ found herself back in Beverly Hills they would renew their friendship. Each morning at 11:00 am Sly would call BJ to see how she was doing. The nurse's were delighted to answer his calls and transfer him to BJ. Sly's voice is most recognizable and very distinctive. His accent is totally "Rocky" even in real life. At 11:00 am on the 4th day, Sly phoned, and the secretary transferred him to BJ's room. However, BJ had checked out early that morning and a new guest was already made comfortable. The new guest answered the phone to hear Sly say, "Good morning, baby, it's Sly, how you doin today?" This guest never stopped talking about her telephone call for the rest of her stay. She was ecstatic that Sly Stallone had actually been on the other end of that phone. I'm sure she is still telling the tale so many years later.

Pothead

I entered the doctor's recovery room to hear Jason cursing the nurses for attempting to put on his pants for discharge. He was a big guy, 230-240 pounds, and not all that tall. He had a tough appearance, one that made you feel that perhaps he was well connected with people you didn't want to get to know. Since he had liposuction of his torso, he was trussed up in a lipo garment (girdle) from his armpits to his knees, a funny site at the least. Being short in the waist, swollen from the surgery, and bound up in that girdle, it was impossible for him to bend at the waist. They were having a difficult time getting him to sit up on the side of the gurney to finish dressing him. He was swearing a bluestreak, yelling for IV Demerol, cursing the doctor because of his pain, and making it as difficult on the staff as possible. Since I don't accept responsibility for Jason until he is in the Shanteque limo, I read the doctor's orders, signed him out on the discharge form, and gathered his belongings. The recovery nurse took me aside and said he usually smoked 4-5 joints a day so they were sending along some Valium. How come that wasn't a surprise, and what made them think he wouldn't continue this little habit during his recuperation.

After another tirade of expletives, Jason was in the wheelchair and on his way to the car. The underground parking garage in this particular medical building is very busy and tight quartered, one lane in, one lane out. The valet quickly pulled up the limo but getting Jason out of the wheelchair and into the backseat was sort of like putting a screaming elephant into a baby carriage. It took ten minutes just to encourage him to stand, none the less turn, put his buttocks on the seat, raise his legs into the car, push himself back on the seat, and then get the seatbelt around him. By the time all of this was accomplished, there were no less than ten cars waiting to exit, and they were none too patient.

All the way to the hotel Jason would say, "Please go slow, please go slow", I was driving 15 miles an hour with cars honking behind me. Suddenly he burst out with, "It's so good not to have breasts anymore." I couldn't help it. Here I was expecting him to pull a 45 on me and instead he makes a comment that simplistic. He then commented on how he was a "real baby" when it came to pain. I phoned ahead and requested that another nurse and a suite attendant meet me in the garage of the hotel. There was no way I was going to extricate Jason from the limo alone. Help soon arrived and Jason was on his way to his room.

A few minutes later he had to "take a piss" as he called it. We managed to assist him to the bathroom and suggested that he "sit" to perform. He informed us that he hadn't "sat" to pee in forty years and wasn't about to now. As a nurse we can only suggest, sure enough, he was midstream when his face paled, his skin grew clammy, his knees buckled and Vesuvius was about to topple. We caught him on the way down, lowered him to the floor, put a cold cloth on his head, elevated his legs, and in 15 seconds his eyes opened. There he was, feet over head, naked on the floor, urine still trickling. How did I get this job. After he was upright he agreed that the next time he would take our advice and "sit" to urinate.

The next day, around noon, I received a call from the bell desk saying one of my guests was in the lobby and had fainted. I grabbed some ammonia and headed on down. I reached the lobby within 20 seconds to find Jason on a bench. He was leaning over with his plumbers crack exposed, in fact half his buttocks was exposed. He had on only his undershorts and lipo garment, needed a shave, and his hair was a mess, what a site. Needless to say there were a few on-lookers. The bellmen helped me put him in a wheelchair. On the way up in the elevator I said, "Jason, you went down to smoke a joint didn't you." He looked up and said, "Yuh," eyes rolling. Just then the joint fell from his hand onto the floor of the elevator. He appeared very groggy and his words were slurred. When he got back to his room his vital signs checked out and he quickly fell asleep. I asked my charge nurse to do a count on his medications. Sure enough, we were 8 short on the Vicodin, Jason had been self medicating. The doctor was notified.

Jason's wife called to see if he was staying another night or coming home. I said he had elected to extend and she sounded relieved. It was evident she did not want to take on his care. She had come to visit him the day before, looked in the room, saw that he was asleep, and left.

Jason woke up 4 hours later, 4 pm., informed the staff he would be leaving, and was escorted to the garage where his ride was to meet him. Jason was by no means physically ready to take on his own care. He insisted on getting in the car and going home. Shanteque is a no smoking facility, since he couldn't smoke his joint in his room, passed out when he went to the lobby, the only recourse for his habit's fulfillment was to take it home. His wife was informed of his intended arrival and his surgeon of his departure.

Shanteque on a Daily Basis

Events transpired on a daily basis at Shanteque that both made me laugh, and rattled my nerves at the same time. In fact, my nerves rattled a lot while at Shanteque. I was responsible for the care and well being of some pretty powerful guests. These people were used to five star hotels and the finest in service. It's true that they were bruised, swollen, under the influence of pain killers and out of their element upon admission. I did have the upper edge the first 24 hours as far as being the one in control of their well being. They, on the most part, were aware of that and quite cooperative. However, once the anesthesia had worn off and they were back in their right mind, outside of painkillers, I had better perform accordingly.

Many events were not worthy of a full chapter but were entertaining in themselves. Like the time many years ago when I had an acid rock star being pushed by a wheelchair into his room. This man had been known to bite off rodents heads during a performance. They did not come any more raucous than this man. I always greeted my guests and went in to make certain all was appropriate. When I approached this guest, still in the wheelchair, I had to take a minute to regain my composure. There he sat in his Mickey Mouse pajamas, thousands of little dime sized red Mickey Mouse heads all over both top and bottoms. He was a delight, quiet, pleasant, and cooperative. Maybe these pajamas were a tribute to those who had lost their heads on stage.

*

The wives of two of L.A.'s most prominent television broadcasting corporation presidents were guests of Shanteque at the same time. Each had undergone facelifts by different doctors and were in rooms at the opposite ends of the hall. Each one had "extremely confidential" written on their reservation card which meant that they both wanted total privacy and confidentiality. No one was to know their beauty was not a God given, everlasting, natural gift. When this happens, everyone tries very hard to respect their wishes. Murphy's Law intercedes man's finest plans. The nurse's complied, my driver made sure their appointments did not conflict so they would not meet at the elevator leaving or arriving, the secretary made certain that all incoming callers used the alias the guest had checked in under. We never admitted to a caller that the individual was at the facility unless the alias name was given. However, that did not prevent both husbands from meeting in the elevator one evening when they both arrived at the same time to visit their wives. Cover blown.

*

I remember the evening that a surgeon visited Shanteque to remove the drains from a guest who had undergone a facelift. He was dressed in a black turtleneck, black jacket, and black pants. This doctor had been under a federal investigation for events involving grand theft, he was still performing surgery, and his patients loved him. He was the shining cosmetic surgeon of the seventies. The assigned nurse followed him into the room with the dressing tray to assist him. Before she had an opportunity to pad the bed with a protective drape, or get the red medical-waste bag opened, the doctor had removed the head dressing and literally whipped the drains out of the patient's head. In so doing the drains had flown up over the doctor's head, spewing blood all over the fabric headboard, wall, bedding, and carpet. He then dropped the drains on the floor, turned and left. I had never witnessed anything so crass or unprofessional. It was apparent to me that he was under the influence of some substance not conducive to good health.

*

A man of mideastern appearance showed up at the retreat accompanied by a beautiful blond American woman. He requested a reservation for his friend for the following Tuesday. When the receptionist checked the reservation book there was no availability for that day, every room had been booked. When told that she was sorry but there were no available rooms, he reached into his pocket and pulled out a roll of bills. He tried to hand the receptionist several $100 dollar bills. She told him that there was no way she could accept the money, that she would be glad to put his friend's name on a waiting list and would call him if there was a cancellation. He became upset, threw the money on the floor, and said that he knew she would find a room by the next day. The young woman told the receptionist to keep the money because he would not take it back. The following morning a cancellation was received, much to the delight of the receptionist. She somehow felt that doom would befall her if she did not perform according to his request.

*

Jocelyn was admitted to the retreat after her facelift. She was accompanied by her boyfriend. He was the smothering kind. He hovered over her and made dictatorial requests of the staff. Do this, did you do that, do you really know what you are doing? It was evident that he was very controlling and did not like to be in a situation in which he knew he was not in control due to ignorance of the situation.

The following morning a man came to the facility and said he was Jocelyn's brother and had some mail for her. He was carrying a manila envelope. The receptionist showed him to Jocelyn's room. Once it was evident which room was Jocelyn's he brushed past the receptionist, went straight into the room, informed Jocelyn that she had been officially served, threw the envelope on her bed, and ran out of the facility.

It turned out he was serving her divorce papers. Jocelyn had been married to a man much older than she was who was now quite ill and in the hospital. Jocelyn had been trying to evade the servicing of the documents as she was hoping the husband would expire prior to any divorce action being initiated. There was a sizeable estate involved.

Jocelyn's boyfriend was furious. He yelled at everyone who entered the room. How could we be so incompetent, why didn't we ask the man for some identification? Somehow the thought arose that perhaps he was upset because he had looked forward to some of the financial rewards Jocelyn may have enjoyed if she had not been served.

*

The charge nurse was administering medications to a middle aged male guest one evening when he became quite personal, asking questions into her private life. He asked her out to dinner to which she declined, she was a married woman. This apparently did not stop him, as the following week she received two dozen long stemmed white roses. A few days later one of the nurses brought in a newspaper article stating he had been arrested for the attempted murder of his girlfriend.

*

One of the nurses was assisting a guest with preparing for discharge. She had undergone a facelift, cheek implant, forehead lift and lip augmentation which left her still quite bruised and swollen. It was certainly noticeable that she had either been

Michael Jackson

Michael was never a guest of Shanteque but he did visit a friend who was staying with us. This was when I was the Administrator of Le Petit Ermitage, the first luxury recovery retreat annexed to L'Ermitage Hotel in Beverly Hills. It was a beautiful European Style two story building fronting Burton Way.

Michael's assistant called me to inform me that Michael would be visiting his friend at Le Petit at 2:00 a.m. the next morning, that the front doors were to be left unlocked for his entry, and that no member of my staff was to be anywhere to be seen during this visitation. He did not want anyone entering our guest's room while he was there, and they were not to be in the hallway during his exit. My staff complied and he came and went in complete privacy.

Porno Queen

Ruby was at the top of her profession. Her body and what she could/would do with it was in world-wide demand. She was queen of the pornography industry and no whips or chains could keep her from busting out all over.

Ruby was only in her 30's but she determined that her face was in need of a bit of tightening. When the buzz of her decision reached certain ears, she was asked if she was willing to have it photographed for a documentary with a twist. Being a porno star she never missed an opportunity to smile for the camera, no matter what the lens angle. She was tall, 5'11" or so, dark long hair, great legs, perfect derriere, and double D's where it counts the most. She carried it all very well. When in full make-up she had the sexy-vixen look, not exactly the girl next door type.

Ruby decided on a full facelift, not that she needed it, most doctors would have told her to go home and come back in 8-10 years. Ruby's line of work can be very tiring and stressful, so many G-string changes etc.

You couldn't help but like Ruby, she had a great personality and wasn't a complainer, the nurses enjoyed caring for her. Her life had been very interesting, taking her all over the world with her pictures published in magazines of all languages. She gave the staff a glossy magazine with hundreds of pictures of herself, whips, chains, feather boas, every angle imaginable. I didn't look at who the publisher was or remember the title. I knew it wasn't exactly the kind of quiet reading material I wanted around the nurse's station so I made sure one of the girls took it home. Ruby was evidently very successful in her industry.

We had been working with the film crew for three days and today was the final filming at Shanteque. The producer's intent for this day was to film her daily routine at Shanteque. The masseuse had dropped by to give her a massage and a little reflexology. They wanted footage of it. The current day's crew composed of the lady producer, the camera man, the sound man, and the masseuse.

We all went to Ruby's room together, she was waiting for us dressed in the wildest animal print silk pajamas. The masseuse helped her out of bed and requested that she change into a bathrobe. The masseuse held up the robe in front of Ruby assuring her of privacy during the disrobing. The producer and I were talking and the film crew was busy filming all the little pretties that decorated the room. Without a moments hesitation, Ruby lightly pushed the robe and the masseuse to the side, and said she had something to show us. We all looked up on time to watch her turn around full front, stark naked. Ruby proudly thrust her chest out and asked us to admire the new breasts that she said her surgeon had given her the year before. She proceeded to comment on how firm and "perky" they were for being so large. She took several steps toward the camera which never stopped rolling. She took a breast in each hand and demonstrated their firmness. She also asked if anyone wanted to feel how natural they were. She didn't have any takers.

I watched the cameraman keep the film rolling, he was not about to miss a flick, the sound man turned crimson, he must have been all of 27 years old, and the producer become pretty in pink, everyone was speechless. I told Ruby they looked great and stepped forward to help her with her robe. I always wondered just where that particular film footage ended up. Just another day at Shanteque.

357 Magnum

Mr. and Mrs. Smith pulled up in front of the retreat in a chauffeur driven stretch limousine. It was quite impressive, a double stretch with personal license plates and what appeared to be a personal driver.

The chauffeur pulled up in front of the hotel and announced their arrival. Mrs. Smith was being admitted on a pre-operative basis and having surgery the next day. Mr. Smith was staying with her throughout her recuperation.

They had reserved the king suite with full patio garden, my favorite suite. It had an original oil painting of two adult swans hanging over the sofa. It was old European in style, heavy gold frame, thick oils with great color blends, a wilderness pond set on a misty morning with swans fluffing their feathers for the start of another day. It was beautiful, perfect for healing.

The room offered a sitting area, buffet with refrigerator and wet bar, and a large king size electric bed set apart in a private alcove. A closet the width of the room was enclosed by glass sliding doors that reflected the crystal chandelier hanging in the middle of the room. It was delightful. A very large marble bath with his and her everything completed this lovely room.

I showed them to their suite, oriented them to the light switches, demonstrated how to call the nurse's station, how to use the phones, gave them their menu to select their evening meal and took their beverage order. Mrs. Smith was around 55 to 60 years old. Mr. Smith was no more than 35. It seemed apparent who held the purse strings. Her diamonds were huge, her shoes Chanel, and her luggage Luis Vuitton, seven pieces of it.

Later that afternoon when I reentered the room I noticed a large bowl of M&Ms on the coffee table and Mrs. Smith was nibbling on them constantly. In the days that followed Mr. Smith kept adding more M&Ms to the dish.

The following morning the nurse entered their room to wake Mrs. Smith for her surgery scheduled for 7:30am. She had a difficult time arousing her. Mrs. Smith seemed in a fog, couldn't remember where she was, and had to be reminded of her impending surgery. The nurse thought she had probably taken a sleeping pill on her own as none had been administered by the staff. Mr. Smith accompanied her to the surgeon's office.

The recovery room nurse called with her pick-up time of 4 pm, giving us the usual hours notice. Our limo picked them up promptly at 4 pm and returned them via the underground private entry. Mrs. Smith was assisted to bed, positioned properly for facial surgery, and surgically assessed. She complained of pain and was medicated according to the doctor's orders with Demerol 75 mg. intramuscularly. This dose will usually give an individual of her size relief of pain and sleep for 3-4 hours. Six hours later Mrs. Smith is still sleeping. Her vital signs were low but not alarming, her color was good, her respirations were even and unlabored. Mr. Smith said that Mrs. Smith never took any medication, and being considered a "lightweight" where medicine was concerned, was probably the reason for her prolonged relief.

Mr. Smith never left her side for the next three days. He was overly involved, always asking what each pill administered was for. He also wanted to make sure she wouldn't run out of pain pills and requested that a refill be obtained before they went home.

On the third day, angry voices were heard coming from their room. They were having an argument, but that was not surprising to the staff. Any two people cooped up in the same room with each other for three days were bound to get on each others nerves. The words money, infidelity, two timer, and gold digger, were overheard by the suite attendant as she cleaned their bathroom. Mrs. Smith used them when she threw her hairbrush at him. She didn't sound that threatening, however, as her speech was still slightly slurred, her movements seemed encumbered, and the hairbrush barely flew five feet. Mr. Smith was not intimidated.

We had called her surgeon to express our concerns about her mental state. The staff had not been administering enough medication to cause this, the doctor should be aware. The doctor requested to see Mrs. Smith at 11:00am that morning.

While they were at the appointment the suite attendant went to make their bed and clean the room. Mr. Smith had draped his bathrobe over a chair and when the maid picked it up to hang it in the closet, a very heavy object fell out of the pocket onto the floor. She took one look at it and went immediately to the nurse's station to tell me what she had found. I followed her back to the suite and she pointed under the chair. It was not a pleasant feeling to see a large black gun laying there. I knew enough to know that it was not a replica even though I knew nothing about guns. I called security to the suite immediately. I thought it better not to handle it myself. I knew that guns had safety mechanisms and I did not know if it was on or off.

What was Mr. Smith up to, who was he, what were his intentions, why a gun at a recovery facility where everyone around had ointment in their eyes, icemasks on their faces, liposuction girdles, head dressings, breast binders, etc., not a very threatening group.

I opened the door to his closet and his duffle was on the floor. Next to the duffle was a plain brown box. I didn't hesitate, I opened the box. It was full of loose M&Ms, not bagged like you would expect to find. For the past three days Mrs. Smith had been nibbling on the M&Ms that Mr. Smith kept replacing in the pretty little glass bowl that had appeared out of nowhere when they were settling into their room the day they arrived. I took a few of the M&Ms and placed them in a baggie.

Security arrived at that point, picked up the gun, and identified it for me, a 357 magnum. He explained the strength of the weapon and how deadly it was. He unloaded it immediately and took down all the information on the owner. I told security I would call him when the Smiths returned so that he could call Mr. Smith, let him know where his gun was, and that it would be returned when he checked out.

When I returned to the nurse's station I called the doctor once again. I told him about the gun and the M&Ms that Mr. Smith kept providing the patient. He asked me to send him some of the candy, I had it delivered to him that afternoon. He, too, was very concerned about Mrs. Smith's lethargy.

The Smiths checked out the next morning. Mr. Smith had cooperated with security regarding the checking of his gun. It was returned to him at the front of the hotel as he was about to enter his limousine.

Ten days later her surgeon called me. He said, "Maggie, can't thank you enough for catching on to the M&Ms and bringing them to my attention." The doctor had sent them out for analysis. Mr. Smith had laced them with a drug that worked like a sedative, would dull her senses to the point that Mr. Smith could control her actions. The doctor had notified the proper authorities and an investigation was in progress.

Extreme Makeover

Shanteque was host to the first fifteen episodes of Extreme Makeover. Originally I had contacted the shows producer, Howard Schultz, offering Shanteque's services in exchange for television coverage of Shanteque on each show. Each patient would receive three days at Shanteque without charge. The usual cost for such a reservation was $1,950.00 at that time. The first seven shows represented a savings to the show of $29,250.00. One of the show's producers contacted me to ask me what I would like to receive in exchange for these services. I asked him what I could have as I had no idea what was customary. I was told I could have visual, audio, named in the credits and a link to Shanteque through the show's website. It all sounded just fine. I was told to put my request in writing.

A few weeks later I received a call from a representative of ABC. They informed me that my requests were excessive and did I realize that ABC receives $186,000.00 for a thirty second commercial. They would make no commitment as to the extent of coverage that Shanteque would receive. I was disappointed as Extreme Makeover had indicated that the coverage was assured and to just name what I would like. I discovered how naive I was to the media world.

One afternoon Howard Schultz walked into my office and sat down. He had stopped by to see one of the patients and I was delighted to have an opportunity to meet him. I asked him how he came to producing Extreme Makeover, what made him think of the concept? He said, "Maggie, I was laying in bed one night, needed a new project, and started thinking about cosmetic surgery. My thoughts evolved into major procedures being performed resulting in extreme transformations and came up with Extreme Makeover." He asked me if I could recommend doctors who were Board Certified and excelled in total body surgeries, not just the face etc. I provided him with several names and was thrilled when I saw Dr. Brent Moelleken and Dr. Robin Yuan being featured on the show. Excellent choices.

The patients started arriving and the nursing care began. Some of the surgeries were ten hours long and 6-7 procedures performed. We were picking up patients at midnight. The patients selected to receive the Extreme Makeovers were delightful individuals, but some of them were hit with a little more than they had anticipated during their first 24 to 48 hours of recuperation. They were swollen, bruised, had drains coming out of various parts of their bodies, injected lips, plastic forms inserted into their cheeks and chins, huge head dressings, liposuction girdles restraining their entire body, their eyes were swollen shut and their nose was packed so they couldn't breathe out of it..

The nursing care began immediately with ice packs, positioning, monitored vital signs, nausea and pain control, vinegar soaks and ointments to the lasered areas, and hours of emotional/psychological support. They were away from family and some had small children, they were in a strange environment, and knew no one. They were physically disabled and totally at the mercy of their care givers. They were in pain and their senses were deprived due to padded head dressings covering their ears and swollen eyes. The patients earned their new looks and the nurses their salaries.

I faithfully watched each episode as it appeared. Shanteque received mention in two of the seven episodes and a visual in two others. It was extremely disappointing.

When the show was picked up for a second season I was again approached by the production company. I now knew just how much nursing care was involved with each patient and that there was no guaranty of TV exposure. I informed the company that I would provide the aftercare for my cost, I would defer any profit. They accepted. I didn't worry about TV exposure at this point, if it happened, it happened.

My biggest joy was watching the episodes as they aired, showing the patients backgrounds, families, and their additional body improvement even after leaving Shanteque. My affiliation with Extreme Makeover was a pleasant experience and a learning opportunity.

Fraud

Jeff made his reservation several months in advance. He was flying in from Florida, was a very successful business man, and had a tight itinerary for life. He was admitted with a nose cast on, swollen and bruised eyes, and a very gentle personality. He had undergone a rhinoplasty. His sister had accompanied him on the trip and shared the room with him. Since his ice mask for his eyes was to be kept cold the nurses were in his room every thirty minutes. This gave them a good opportunity to get to know them well. The two were dedicated to each other. Janet, his sister, was planning surgery herself in the near future and was happy to get to know the nurses and routines so she would be more in tune to Shanteque when it was her turn.

Jeff stayed for two days, his swelling was beginning to subside, the packing had been removed, he could breathe, and he had regained his strength. The only treatment at this point was to sleep with his head elevated, keep ice to his eyes, and continue taking his antibiotic until it was gone. He was ready to go to his private hotel room.

Six months later Janet joined us as a guest at Shanteque, she had her breasts enhanced and her nose revamped too. Everyone was delighted to see each other again and her recuperation was uneventful. This time Jeff accompanied her.

Two years later I received a request from an attorney in Florida for a copy of both Janet's and Jeff's final bills, copy of the credit card receipt, and the reservation cards they had signed. They enclosed a subpoena for these requests. I was curious but soon forgot all about it.

Another two years passed and yet another subpoena arrived requesting my presence in a Florida courtroom for the following week. Shanteque was booked solid for that week. It takes months for me to plan an escape from the business. I need to find Administrative nurses to take my place. I phoned the prosecuting attorney and told him of my dilemma. I asked him what Jeff was being prosecuted for. I was informed that he was the head of the largest credit card fraud ring the FBI had ever uncovered. That all Shanteque expenses as well as surgeon fees had been paid for with fraudulent credit cards. He needed me to verify that the Shanteque statements were indeed authentic, that Jeff had been a guest of Shanteque, and that the copy of our registration card was indeed ours. I requested a later court date and a few days later he called me back and said that the defense said they would accept the documents as authentic without my personal verification. I did not have to make the trip. I was delighted.

The Lament of the Lipo Girdle

Many of you have had liposuction and know the lament of the liposuction girdle. It's like being trussed back into the uterus with no way to pee. The girdles are tight (in order to be affective), binding (because your body swells around the leg/arm holes and also the pudendal areas), dirty (because you continue to seep fluids for 24 hours), and sometimes smelly (because as a woman it's doggone hard to pee in a straight line with one on), and perspiration is always a factor.

We tried everything at Shanteque to help our guests handle the disadvantages of wearing a girdle. It may have been a chest girdle for a man undergoing Gynecomastia surgery (removal of excess fat in breast area) or a woman with a various number of breast procedures. Usually it was a full body girdle from the waist to the ankles with full side zips.

Swelling of the extremities occurs because the fluids are being forced there due to the stricture of tissues caused by the tightness of the girdle. Often the nurses would have to unlatch the girdles to replace reinforcement dressings over the cannula insertion sites. The use of Tumescent liposuction, (inserting saline prior to sucking fat) lends to a 24 hour period of seepage of the saline and small amounts of body fluids. This can be quite messy if not addressed before hand. Rule number one, pad your bed well or stay overnight in a recovery retreat that prepares the bed for this dilemma. The challenge after reinforcing the dressings was to re-latch/zip the girdle. The trick with the full side zips was to latch all the hook and eyes first, then attempt to raise the zipper. This sometimes took two if not three nurses. The staff would then place icepacks in strategic locations to help with the swelling, offer as much emotional support as possible and encouragement not to lose faith in their decision to have undergone the procedure.

At least a man could still stand and urinate normally, defecation was another matter for both sexes. Women had the hardest time. The girdles never seemed to be put on straight, it's difficult to align a girdle properly when it is put on the body after surgery. The patient is still anesthetized, the body is a dead weight, and you just try your best to get it in place. That leaves it up to the nurse, post-operatively, to do her best in re-aligning it so the patient can urinate without soaking herself. The hole in the girdle, structured for urination, is a small oval area, usually requiring to be cut larger. The nurses found that placing an emesis basis (kidney shaped basin used when nauseous) between the legs sometimes worked out perfectly. Nurses are great improvisers.

Walking is the key to recovery with liposuction. After laying in bed all night, swelling has set in. It's painful to get out of bed and more painful to start walking. However, if you don't, your recovery will take twice as long and you certainly don't want the risk of blood clots.

The more you walk, the easier it gets. It's the muscles that tighten down on the surrounding tissues as you walk that stimulates circulation and that, in return, removes the swelling.

If the above has not deterred you, and I hope it has not, I want you to know that I have not met anyone who was not delighted with their results thirty days down the line.

Las Vegas Loser

I received a phone call from a Mr. H. He said a very dear friend of his was having a cosmetic surgical procedure and he wanted her to stay at Shanteque. She had been planning on going directly home but he felt she needed the care, pampering, and medical observation that she would receive from our nurses. He had heard about Shanteque and it's wonderful care and wanted her to experience it. He thought she should stay a minimum of two nights. He provided me with the name, address, and phone number of Cassandra, his friend, and his credit card information with direct instructions that whatever she wanted was to be placed against this card. I remember thinking, "Why can't I find someone as thoughtful and considerate of my well-being." A true gentleman.

A confirmation letter was sent to Cassandra. I had the opportunity to speak with her prior to admission. She informed me that Mr. H. was not the one true love of her life and she had informed him of it. He was aware that the relationship was one sided but he wanted to do this for her anyway. She had tried to talk him out of it, not wanting to be indebted to him for this amount, but he had insisted, "friend to friend" he said.

I had a minimum of two more conversations with Mr. H. He called to verify that her reservation was indeed on our books, and that I would not forget our previous conversations which included my personal promise to oversee her care. I reassured him that all was in order and, "No, I had not forgotten our conversation."

The day of Cassandra's admission arrived. I had never seen such a beautiful, groggy person. With no makeup, 4 hours of anesthesia on board, pain killers swimming around in her veins, blond tangled hair about her face, and tight dressings around her chest, she was still one of the loveliest women I had ever seen.

The following day I made rounds as usual and when I reached Cassandra's room she was sitting upright in bed, alert and smiling. I sat down at the table at the foot of the bed and the warmth of her personality rendered a very easy, comfortable conversation to ensue. She commented on how wonderful the staff was, how comfortable and secure she felt at Shanteque. She loved the food served from the hotel kitchen. She went on to tell me that she had been a stewardess when she met a wonderful older man whom she later married. He had shown her a privileged life as he was financially well off. She made the comment that he treated her as a precious possession and she became stifled. The marriage ended and she was now trying to put the pieces back together in her life. She had not planned on recuperating at Shanteque as the funds were limited. She needed to have her breast implants replaced, it was a medical decision, not a personal one.

She continued to explain that she had met Mr. H. through a friend and he had been quite smitten with her. He purchased expensive gifts to impress her. She had returned a very expensive blouse and wanted to return a gorgeous fur coat. Mr. H. would not take no for an answer. He was an entrepreneur in the investment business and he traveled extensively about the world, his home was in Las Vegas.

Later that day Mr. H. visited her. He appeared very nice, attentive to her needs. He commented on how grateful he was to Shanteque for taking such good care of her.

Cassandra later informed me that he was irritated that she had received a bouquet of long stemmed red roses from a friend. Mr. H. knew he had not sent them, although his floral arrangement was larger and in center stage on the table in the middle of the room.

The following day he returned, Cassandra was due to check out that morning. She was not feeling that strong yet, and after a discussion, he agreed that she should remain an additional two days. Cassandra was delighted. This had impressed her as he truly seemed to want to meet her needs.

However, the following day Mr. H. arrived for his regular visit to find another man in her room. It was someone who she was dating, a new relationship, nothing heavy. They were talking, not holding hands or showing displays of affection. Mr. H. was extremely upset, this was his territory. He left Shanteque and flew back to Las Vegas.

Cassandra went home the following morning as scheduled, having incurred a bill in excess of $4100.00. This amount was placed against Mr. H's credit card as we had his signature on Cassandra's reservation card.

Two months later I received correspondence from VISA stating that Mr. H. was not going to honor this charge. I was caught by surprise, $4100.00 dollars was a pretty large sum of money to a small business. I wrote VISA and explained the circumstances of this reservation and that I had his signature on file. They informed me that without his signature on the charge slip itself, they could not require him to pay.

I spoke with Cassandra about Mr. H's actions and she was devastated that he would do such a thing. She was not in a financial position to pay the bill and I did not ask her to. I mentioned that the portion of her bill from the hotel for her room was $900.00.

A few weeks later I received a call from a man asking if I would be in my office later that day. I said yes and he said he wanted to meet with me regarding Cassandra's bill. I had no idea what he meant by that, but knew I would soon find out and my curiosity was peaked. He sounded like a "take charge" kind of guy.

At 5 pm a very good looking man, someone I could certainly see Cassandra endeared to, came to my office. He was tall, had a great mustache, warm expressive eyes, a certain amount of rustic charm about him combined with a cool casual clothing style. He said he had been talking to Cassandra and she was totally distraught about Mr. H's behavior. She had loved her stay at Shanteque and the nurses were wonderful. She was embarrassed and humiliated and he could not allow that to continue. He was amazed at the gaul of the man to place her in this position. He was there to give me the $900.00 to take care of the hotel portion.

I was truly touched by this man's generosity and desire to give Cassandra some peace over this matter. He asked that I not give her his name but to let her know the bill had been satisfied. He then gave me the money and left.

I didn't have to tell Cassandra who paid the bill, she knew immediately.

From Chantique to Shanteque

HISTORY OF FRAUD AND EMBEZZLEMENT

It was 1993 and Le Petit Ermitage, the first exclusive cosmetic surgery aftercare facility in Beverly Hills, had been closed due to the owner losing the host hotel to bankruptcy. The bankruptcy was not affiliated to the failure or success of Le Petit, but to the numerous other hotels owned and over leveraged. The L' Ermitage was in Chapter 11 when I joined the nursing staff of Le Petit in 1987, it just took the banks another six years for the final foreclosure. I had been a Charge Nurse for four years and the Administrator for three years prior to its closing. I knew the business inside out. The doctors were all familiar with me and my staff and we were comfortable with the way we each did business. Aftercare had been firmly established as a requirement of most major surgeons if they performed a facelift or multiple procedures on a patient. Prior to aftercare retreats, patients went home. The risk of complications was extensive when there were no medical personnel around to assist patients with ambulating, check drains for proper functioning, administer injectable pain/ nausea medications, assess the surgical areas and assure proper food/fluid intake.

With the final closing of Le Petit's doors, which was done without notice when the sheriff showed up and posted the final notice on the front door, a large void was left in the aftercare business. I pondered my professional future for several months and came to the realization that the one area I loved and knew the most about, was aftercare. The doctors had been calling me to assist them with obtaining nurses for private duty care for their patients during this time. They all wanted another retreat to be made available.

I knew that my doctors would return to my support if I opened my own retreat. The only stumbling block at this time, February of 1994, was the financial backing. I decided to advertise for a financial backer and placed an ad on a Friday in the Beverly Hills Courier, it was small and simple: RN seeks financial backing to establish cosmetic surgery aftercare retreat.

The paper had not been on the streets two hours when I received a call from Mr. T. It was a brief conversation during which he wanted to know how much ownership I expected if he and his partner, Mr. C, were to finance the business. This threw me because I had not really thought that far as yet. Never having been in this position, and feeling that the money was the major risk factor, I said 25%. He said 15% was the norm, we settled on 20%. I later learned how unjust this split truly was. I had undervalued what I was bringing to the table: the following of all local surgeons, a full staff of specialized nurses, and my expertise of seven years in the business, (we opened with over 100 reservations on the books).

Mr. T. requested a meeting which was set up for the following week. I chuckled to myself when I first saw them, a total replica of Laurel and Hardy. Mr. C. said he had been looking for a business for his wife and that she would be the owner, he would be the hands-on partner. Mr. T. said that unfortunately, he had been placed in a questionable tax shelter by his accountant, and was under an IRS investigation. His share of the business would also go to Mrs. C. for the time being. When the investigation was done, Mrs. C. would transfer the stock to Mr. T., they had been business partners and very good friends for many years. I didn't have reason to question this at the time. We discussed the business, I showed them numerous articles, stories, etc. on Le Petit Ermitage and myself, and must have appeared quite credible, as they told me to find a host hotel and arrange a meeting with the manager.

I learned of a hotel that had just been renovated called the Beverly Prescott, located at the corner of Beverly Drive and Pico Blvd., only a few blocks south of Beverly Hills. The location was perfect, I made an appointment with the General Manager for the following day. The G.M. met with me and expressed his interest in establishing a relationship. His dad was a doctor and he knew the value that a business such as this could provide to a hotel. The patients, half of which came from out of town, would book reservations in the main hotel for their pre-operative days and then transfer back to the hotel for an additional 5-7 days after their stay at the recovery retreat. It was a perfect blend. We set up a meeting for Mr. T., Mr. C, and myself for the next day.

The meeting was successful, we reached a meeting of the minds on the rent to be charged to Chantique for the use of the entire 6th floor. I moved into one of the rooms the following week to oversee the construction of the nurse's station, kitchenette, and utility area. Toilets were removed from two bathrooms and capped. A shampoo basin was installed in one of the bathrooms, as well as storage for supplies. The other bath was converted into a kitchenette. A platform was placed over the tubs and shelving units installed above. Countertops and cupboards were custom designed for the nurse's station. It was efficient, attractive, and very functional. The second bath came from a room used as my office. A sleeper couch was purchased for my office for the early morning admits for patients that had surgery the day before, and had remained in the surgeon's recovery room over night. Our rooms were full Tuesday through Thursday. Since check-out time was not until 11 am, we needed someplace to hold these early birds.

In six weeks we were operational. A cocktail party was held on the roof of the hotel in a beautiful panoramic party room. It was attended by our referring surgeons and their staffs. Everyone came, as Chantique had been anxiously anticipated.

For the first 6 weeks of operation I spent 12 to 14 hour days, seven days a week, at Chantique. Some of the staff was new and had to find out what worked and what didn't work in methods of doing their daily routines of guest care, how to work with one another most effectively, how to relate with the different departments of the hotel, i.e. bellmen, housekeeping, room service, valet. It was a learning process for everyone. When the business is your own, and you're a nurse, you feel completely responsible for the care and satisfaction that your guests receive. I could not bring myself to leave until most of my guests had been prepared for their night's sleep. I soon learned I had to let go a little to maintain my own health and equilibrium.

Four months passed uneventfully. Business was flourishing, reservations were flowing in, the staff was adjusting to the new work environment and all was wonderful. Mr. C. stopped by every day to pick up the discharged guest folios showing their total bill and method of payment. The checks and cash were part of this collection. The agreement we had made was that I was in charge of the administration, hiring, staffing, public relations, advertising, media, and nursing care. Mr. T. and Mr. C. were in charge of bill payment, record keeping, purchases of large items like refrigerators, etc. They were to have their bookkeeper, Miss K, keep the books and give me a statement at the end of each month so I could be kept abreast of the financial status of the corporation.

At the beginning of the fifth month, Mr. C. came into my office and sat down. He had a very serious expression on his face and I knew that something was amiss. He informed me that Mr. T. was no longer a partner, that I was not to talk to him as he was not to be allowed on the property. I was shocked. When I asked what had happened, I was informed that Mr. T. had never given Mr. C. any money towards the original start-up investment. He said Mr. T had asked Mr. C. to put up his share for him, which Mr. C. said that he had done. Mr. C. said that he and Mr. T. had a disagreement and that Mr. C. had changed his mind about the loan. It was no longer a loan, the corporation was now 80% Mrs. C.'s and 20% mine. I told Mr. C. that he could not do that, that a lawsuit was inevitable and that as far as I was concerned Mr. T. was still a partner. I had not had a disagreement with Mr. T., and I would not cut myself off from him as requested.

I called Mr. & Mrs. T. later that evening. They told me that they had given Mr. C. a check for $45,000.00. I asked to see a copy of the check, please, just show me some proof of payment. None was ever offered. Within six months the corporation was served with a lawsuit claiming ownership by Mr. T. The next three years were spent in and out of depositions and court appearances. It was during this time that I learned that the two had previously been business partners in a hard-money lending business with several offices in southern California. It was my understanding that they would borrow money from individual investors, make high risk loans at healthy interest rates, and when the loans were satisfied (paid off) they would retain the funds instead of paying the investors back. It was rumored that they did this to the tune of over $20,000,000.00.

Mr. T. had turned states evidence against Mr. C., and that was when Mr. C. shut Mr. T. out of our corporation. At the conclusion of the lawsuit, Mr. T. was awarded a judgement of close to $300,000.00.

During our third and final year at the Beverly Prescott, Mr. T. started paying the rent late, and at times, not at all. The general manager had now changed, the new manager sized Mr. C. up immediately. Although the monthly statements provided me indicated that all rents had been paid, they had not. We were given notice by the hotel that our lease would not be renewed. It was at that time I learned that Chantique was $50,000.00 in arrears to the hotel.

However, God works in mysterious ways. Since we were leasing the entire floor for a year at a time, we should not have been charged the room tax which we had been paying. Mr.

C. took this fact to the city of L.A. and a ruling was passed down that Mr. C. was right. The city owed a refund of over $50,000.00 for the previous three years. Mr. C. came back from the final meeting rejoicing at the fact that he would be receiving this check. HOWEVER, since it was the hotel who had been paying the tax to the city, the city returned the check for $50,000.00 to the hotel. Naturally, the hotel kept the money in lieu of the unpaid rent.

Once Mr. T's. lawsuit was served, Mr. C. took it upon himself to close out the Chantique corporation so that Mr. T. could not have access to additional income generated by the company. He renamed the business Le Palais Chantique and moved it to the Century Plaza Hotel. I learned of the new corporation formation six weeks after the fact. Mr C. said he had gone to Nevada to form the new corporation. Once we moved to the Century Plaza, I was informed that Mrs. C. was going to be placed on the payroll for $5000.00 a month. I had not been given a vote in that decision. She did come in every once and a while to answer phones and drive patients to their doctor's appointment.

The move to the Century Plaza took place in January of 1997. It was an ideal arrangement. The hotel's configuration offered a very long hallway that we partitioned at each end, leasing 23 rooms. The rent was $62,000.00 a month. Business was excellent and as the months went by I was presented with a monthly statement by Mr. C's accountant, always indicating all creditors were satisfied. I had been assured that statements would be accurate, no further misrepresentation.

One year later, at 8:00 am in the morning, I was delivered a letter from the hotel's accounting department. Chantique was to satisfy the outstanding rent in the amount of over $300,000.00 by 5:00 pm, or we were to cease and desist our operation. I was in shock. How could this be, my statements had always indicated that the rent had been paid. I confronted Mr. & Mrs. C. who had no excuses to offer. Mr. C. disappeared that afternoon and returned with a letter for the hotel indicating that he had placed Chantique in Chapter 11. This was his solution to the problem. Tie the hands of the hotel as they could not throw us out of the hotel if a Chapter 11 exists. During the next few months I continued to function, but never knew if we would exist by the end of each day.

It was during this time that I asked to see the bankruptcy documents. I wanted to see how I had been named, but my name did not appear anywhere. I asked Mrs. C. why my name was not listed as an owner on the documents. I was informed that I was not an owner, that she was 100% owner of Le Palais Chantique. I then realized that they had also defrauded me of my ownership in the corporation, which in the end worked to my benefit.

About ten months into the Chapter 11 filing, Mrs. C. told me that Mr. C. would not be coming in that day, he was not feeling well. This continued for the next two days. On the third day she took me aside and informed me that Mr. C. had been arrested and was incarcerated. She did not know when he would be back in civilization. I later discovered the charges were embezzlement from previous business partners. Why didn't it surprise me.

I eventually learned that in one months time the Chapter 11 would expire. The hotel would then be free to immediately require Le Palais Chantique to cease and desist operations. I wrote a letter to our surgeons informing them that Chantique would be closing as of a specific date but Mrs. C. refused to allow me to mail it. She did not intend to inform the doctors of the closing of Chantique. I informed her that we could not continue to accept reservations knowing we would not be operational. She said if we informed them, they would immediately start using alternative facilities, she wanted every reservation she could get until the day she closed. I informed her that I could not be a part of that deception. People were planning their surgeries and aftercare was a major part of their recuperation.

I would not have them finding out the day before their surgery that they would not have a facility to recuperate in.

I gave Mrs. C. my resignation and was told to make it immediate. I was also informed to leave my car keys on her desk before I left. I was driving an automobile leased by the corporation.

I then found myself, with my cardboard box of belongings, taking a cab home from a corporation I had started, and worked so very hard to build for four years. It was a comical situation, but I don't let life's little trials hold me down for long. When one does not have wheels, the fact that one does not have a job is of no consequence. The next morning I got up at my usual time, walked across the street to the only car dealership at my end of town, Mercedes Benz, and bought a Mercedes. I'd always wanted one.

Mrs. C. took my place as the Administrator of Chantique. She knew nothing of running a recovery retreat, zero about nursing, and the only accounting she was familiar with were her credit cards at Neimans and Saks. She and her husband had just destroyed a business that my staff had made a very good living at for the past four years. She was not the staff's favorite person. Several resigned immediately, knowing disaster was eminent.

I wrote a letter to my surgeons and their patient consultants, informing them that I was no longer the Administrator of Le Palais Chantique. I did not want them holding me responsible for whatever might ensue. During the following weeks Mrs. C. sold off the assets of the corporation.

My next stop was to the attorney that had represented Mr. T. in his lawsuit against Chantique. Since he knew Mr. & Mrs. C. and all aspects of the business, I wanted him to take my case. I wanted to sue them for stealing the corporation and embezzling what turned out to be hundreds of thousands of dollars in corporate funds. Mr. K. accepted my case, having first obtained permission from Mr. T. to represent me.

Permission was required because he would be using information he had obtained while retained by Mr. T. I also had to agree to pay Mr. T. 30% of whatever rewards I should receive.

I will jump ahead in time and tell you that for the next six years we were in and out of the court room. Mr. C. never did appear, even though he had been released from jail prior to completing his four year term. He had Mrs. C. appear. Mrs. C. was on her third attorney by the sixth year. The court ruled that the statute of limitations had expired on the first three years that we were in business, I could only lay claim to losses incurred in the fourth year. Most of the theft had occurred during the first three years, so my judgment was minimal to my loss. By the time the attorneys received 40%, and Mr. T. 30%, I received a check for a nominal amount.

Getting back to October of 1998, having just resigned from Le Palais Chantique, I knew I had to lay a master plan for the next ten years of my life. My parents had both passed away in 1995 leaving me an inheritance. Should I risk some of this money and start my own retreat once more, or should I do private duty nursing or get a job in a surgeon's office and play it safe. I don't know why I asked myself these questions, being a Leo lady, I knew very well I would forge ahead and begin again.

The economy was still doing well, so the hotels weren't hungry for tenants requiring discounted rooms. However, I did locate a very cute boutique hotel in West Hollywood named Le Montrose. We negotiated a lease and Shanteque was born. Since I had brought the name "Chantique" to the table in 1994, I wanted to retain it. I knew the spelling would have to be changed, but I could keep the phonetics. Chantique became Shanteque.

In March of 1999 my staff quickly and loyally returned, delighted to learn that I now had my very own business, no investors. It was frightening for me. If it did not work, if the reservations did not come in and I could not meet overhead and salaries, it could cost me my entire savings. I experienced more than one sleepless night. I remember what my dad had told me,

"You can't win if you don't play the game." I don't think he knew that I would be playing the game with his money. I also knew that if I didn't take this risk I would never know if I could have made it.

The reservations did come in, my previous referral surgeons all returned. We were in the black from the first month we opened. There were several months when I had to reduce my own salary in order to meet expenses but the census continued to grow and we were soon a very viable business again.

Eighteen months later, at the end of my lease at Le Montrose, I was able to negotiate a lease with Le Meridien Hotel for a private wing. This would bring us closer to Beverly Hills. It also gave us a Beverly Hills address, even though we were in the half of the hotel that was in Los Angeles. The main half of the hotel lay over the line into Beverly Hills. Le Meridien was one block away from my apartment and next door to the Mercedes dealership from which I had purchased my Mercedes two years before. It was a perfect location and business continued to thrive. The staff grew, the census rose, and suddenly it was September 11th, 2001. The country stood still, numb, disbelieving, vulnerable. I kept waiting for Los Angeles to be targeted. I couldn't believe that with our population there wasn't a plan to attack LA. I went to work as usual. I didn't know how this would affect business. I felt that if I lived on the East coast I would not get on an airplane to fly to Los Angeles to get a facelift. In the next ten days we took 28 cancellations, mostly from people that would have had to fly in. The industry saw a definite slowdown, but it was brief. I truly believe that people soon took a turn in their thinking. They began to feel that if they had a short time to live, or were going to live in fear, they were going to do it with a new face or new body. I also feel that they no longer were saving for their retirement, they were going to spend it while they were able to enjoy the results. Business soon prospered once more.

In 2002, Extreme Makeover hit the television screen. Shanteque had taken care of the first 20 patients, ten shows, and were renewed for a second year. Multiple procedures, performed at one time, burst upon the scene. These patients had literally been taken off the farm, had four to six cosmetic surgical procedures performed, and were not always prepared for the recovery period. They required extensive emotional reinforcement from the staff as well as nursing care. They were all lovely individuals, extremely grateful for the opportunity they were experiencing, and appreciative of the care given. I loved watching the program when it aired and seeing my patients emerge with their new bodies. How thrilled and happy they were. I knew their lives would never be the same, only better.

The following year The Swan and Nip and Tuck were added to our viewing pleasure. Cosmetic surgery was now front page news. Shanteque was over flowing into the hotel's regular rooms.

In 2005, Shanteque was a thriving business. Two lovely ladies approached me in April of this year expressing their interest in purchasing Shanteque. They asked me what price I would like to receive, I told them my price, they accepted the terms, and I am now retired and sharing my story with you.

Section II

Attacking Grandmother Nature

Fighting Grandmother Nature

I don't like to blame the aging process on Mother Nature. After all, she gives us the flowers that bloom, the sun that shines, and the birds that sing. I prefer to think of it as Grandmother Nature who comes sneaking in the back door with her aging bag of tricks. She doles them out along life's path, through the decades of our lives.

Your twenties are marvelous, your skin is firm, your complexion is perfect. Your breasts are perky, your buttocks sits perfectly beneath you. Your closest thought to cosmetic surgery is the removal of a wart from your index finger. You never think of your navel because it's tucked ever so neatly up into your diaphragm. Taught eyelids are to be blended and stroked with brilliant colors to accentuate their depth and mysticism. Skin care is comprised of washing your face in the morning because you forgot to take off your make-up the night before.

Your mouth turns up when you smile and your eyes sparkle, there's not a wrinkle or sag on the horizon. Life is perfect, it's fun, it's beautiful, and so are you!

The thirties add milestones... a home, children, and a husband with equal demands. At this point in life the tummy has stretch marks, the breasts have stretch marks, and the pocket book has stretch marks. There's just no time or money for self-pampering. A bubble bath is a luxury.

Throughout these years, however, you do manage to shave your legs routinely and get in a few "rays" to keep a bronze tone to your skin. You shave your legs because, heaven forbid, you should crawl into the marital bed with "stubble", and the "sun" is an hour or two of self-indulgence, stolen when time permits.

Before you know it the forties have snuck in the back door. The children are in college, the husband is either an "ex", asleep on the couch, never home from the office, or on the golf course.

You now have time to start taking a good look at your own body. You wonder what the original color of your hair was before Grandmother Nature took over with those dull earthtones. Your neck has never looked worse. If you were a heavy smoker or a sun-goddess your neck now looks like a cross between brown crackled glass and alligator skin. Your chin is starting to flap back at you in the mirror, and your eyes appear lost in the folds of your lids. Your breasts droop, your tummy sags, and your face is starting to look like a road map. The worse part is you don't feel a day older than you did in your twenties.

It's time to sprinkle a little spice on your life. This chapter is to let you know there is an answer. It addresses the woman who wants to maintain her physical appearance as long as possible through cosmetic surgery, in other words, wage war with Grandmother Nature. Women I know want to continue to look as vital on the outside as they feel on the inside.

Let's Get Started

Before considering cosmetic surgery, it's important to lose any excess pounds you've been collecting over the years, and break the smoking habit if it exists. Smoking is one of the greatest contributors to the aging process. Inhalation puckers your lips and creates multiple vertical ridges between lip line, and nostrils. These ridges provide great runways for your lipstick to race out beyond your natural lip line as if sucked up into your nostrils. Smoking also contracts small blood vessels and inhibits circulation. Many cosmetic surgeons will not operate on heavy smokers. Most will require the patient to stop smoking two weeks prior to surgery and continue to refrain from smoking for ten days post-operatively. The incidence of complications after cosmetic surgery is much higher with smokers versus non-smokers. This is due to the fact that the development of new collateral circulation (tiny little blood vessels) is jeopardized by the long range damage of heavy smoking. Smoking yellows your teeth, disenchants your breath, and costs money that could better be spent on a relaxing, soothing, cleansing facial. The color of your teeth may not seem of major concern to you at this point in time, but as we continue to improve your body, your teeth will become a focal point of your beautiful new face, and will take on new meaning.

The aging process also depends on the amount of sun one has received in his/her lifetime and the genetic factor. Genes and the Sun God are two major enemies of aging gracefully. The sun's ultra-violet rays dehydrate the skin, removing valuable water from cells and tissues. This results in a toughening of the epidermis (top layer of the skin) and as the years pass the damage accumulates, resulting in a leathery appearance. You might say the sun sucks the moisture out of your skin, as a prune drying on the bush.

Genetics play a very important role in determining your muscle tone, skin elasticity, lifespan of the collagen layer, and longevity of your natural hair color. Cosmetic aging that is correctable with cosmetic surgery is due to the weakening of the body's collagen layer, causing wrinkles.

Eyelid Surgery

(BLEPHAROPLASTY)

The eyes are usually the first to divulge the passing of the years. Fat pads can collect beneath the lower lids causing a puffy, early-morning, unsightly appearance. The upper lids start to sag and a condition called "creeping" (for lack of a better descriptive word) sets in. At this point you have to hold one edge of the eyelid taught so you can apply your eye make-up without getting the tie-dye effect. Crinkling initially takes place at the outer edges of the eyes, it then begins its major invasion of the upper and lower orbital area. Now is when you start to feel just the slightest twinge of emotional depression when facing the mirror. This just can't be happening. You don't feel any different than when you were younger, but the image reflected certainly is.

It's time to consider a "blepharoplasty" or eyelid surgery. This is probably one of the simplest of cosmetic surgical procedures. The incision for the upper eyelid usually lies in the natural crease of the lid and is visible only when the eye is shut. Ask your surgeon exactly where the suture line will be placed and just how far outside of the natural fold it will extend, if necessary to do so. If there is a serious collection of wrinkles on the outer perimeters of the eyes it may be necessary for the suture line to be extended in order to remove as many of these wrinkles as possible.

It is also interesting for you to ask whether the incision line will be closed with sutures, or a relatively new method of gluing the incision together. The suture lines disappear slowly over the next several months to blend into the natural curve of the lid. The only usual giveaway is if make-up is allowed to collect along this line. Blot your eye make-up well.

Lower eyelid surgery is also a simple procedure. Some surgeons are now able to remove unsightly fat pads from beneath the eye without the need for an incision. The fat pads are cut out from behind the lid. If the problem is excess skin and an incision is required, it is generally placed just below the lash line, making it virtually undetectable. Skilled surgeons are very careful not to disrupt the existing eyelashes.

Recuperation is seven to ten days. The immediate post-op care is ice compresses through the first night to prevent swelling and bruising. These can be continued for three to four days as they will not only feel soothing, but will assist in the reduction of the swelling. Warm compresses can safely be started on the fourth day. This increases the circulation to the eye area and helps clear away the dead blood cells causing discoloration.

A good rule-of-thumb is no eye make-up until twenty-four hours after the sutures have been removed. This allows the suture holes to heal thoroughly and avoids infection when eye make-up is once again applied. Purchase new eye make-up and applicators to verify they will be as bacteria-free as possible.

Forehead Lift

(CORONAL)

The forehead also exhibits telltale signs around the same time as the eyes. It starts to furrow horizontally and then the vertical frown lines set in between the eyes. This area is called the glabella and squinting plays a large part in the development of these lines.

The surgery to address the forehead furrows is called a "Coronal" or "Forehead Lift". This surgery not only removes the horizontal "trenches" across the forehead but raises the eyebrows and gives a much more youthful appearance to the eyes. The squinting muscle can also be cut so the vertical lines don't reappear. This smoothes the area and removes two additional adornments of maturity.

The placement of the suture line is generally one and a half to two inches behind the hairline extending from ear to ear. It may sound unsightly at this time, but with the cosmetic closure that is performed, the incision mingles into the roots of the hair and can be easily camouflaged by a new hairdo or a small amount of "teasing" at the root line.

A pressure head dressing is applied after the surgery to assist in the approximation of the suture line and prevent bleeding. Swelling of the forehead and eyes may be involved post-operatively so lay with your head elevated on two or three pillows. Apply cold compresses to your forehead and eyes for the first twenty-four to forty-eight hours. Metal clips or "staples" may be used for the closure. Half of these, or every other clip, will be removed around the fourth day, with the remainder removed two days later. This is due to the tension that is placed on the suture line and as an added precaution that you will have a well approximated closure.

Seven to ten days should be removed from your social calendar for this procedure. This will allow your suture line to heal well enough for your hair to be styled, and for any residual bruising and swelling to dissipate. Do not color or perm your hair for six weeks post-operatively as these chemicals are very caustic to your suture line. You may shampoo your hair two days post-operatively but use only the pads of your fingers and not your fingernails. Be very careful when combing or brushing out your hair that you do not "snag" a staple. You may have to play with a new hair style for a while due to the small amount of hair loss, however, you will have a wonderful time applying creative make-up to your new eyebed (that area of eye that had previously disappeared under your fallen eyebrows).

Since some hair is lost with the 1/2 to one inch of scalp that is removed, your surgeon will determine your candidacy for this procedure. The present height of your forehead is also a factor. If your forehead is already very high you do not want to pull it back another inch. Your scalp will feel numb for several months but the sensation does return, a small inconvenience when compared to the positive results the surgery offers.

Facelift

(RHYTIDECTOMY)

The next area of the body to exhibit aging is the chin and neck. How much the neck/chest area ages depends extensively on how many pleasurable moments you indulged in worship of the Sun Goddess in your earlier years. Many women lose their chin line at an early age due to heredity. It either exhibits itself as a true double chin via excess skin and fat, or as a flap of skin that actually hangs down as an appendage beneath their chin. In other words, the turkey has begun to gobble.

Your cheeks may have begun to sag, your mouth definitely turns down at the corners, and your collagen layer is at half-mast. You have found yourself heading for the turtle-neck counter in the stores and your plunging necklines have found their way to the back of the closet. No way are you planning on drawing attention to this part of your body.

There is an answer and it's called the Facelift. I know you're all familiar with it. You've heard it mentioned in jest, ridiculed, used as focal points in comedy skits, and gossiped about over the bridge table, but I feel fairly certain you haven't heard this factual story. One of my guests at Le Petit Ermitage told me she had included a facelift in her divorce agreement because, as she put it, "That man put about 100,000 miles on this chassis and by damn he's going to pay for the retread!"

The facelift, sometimes in combination with a neck lift, is one of the most exciting cosmetic surgical procedures to experience. The results are right out there for everyone to see and admire so they can tell you just how terrific you look.

Cosmetic surgery is a personal choice, and whether a woman wants to divulge the fact that she has undergone the procedure is completely up to her. If a facelift is completed while still in the 45 - 55 age range the results are less dramatic and the new-you can still be attributed to your 'new interest in exercise, proper eating habits, and a few weeks at a spa.' It is not always necessary to divulge your surgery to others, this is your choice. The placement of suture lines are now such that it is very difficult to visualize whether or not surgery has taken place.

An important question to ask your surgeon is whether or not he places a suture line in front of, or behind, the trucus. The trucus is the small protrusion from your cheek into the front of the ear. A suture line skillfully placed behind the trucus is much less visible. Look at his "after" pictures to make sure the trucus remains evident. It's also important to note that there will be two suture lines on the side of your scalp causing some hair loss. This is inevitable with a full lower facelift with symmetrical results. Beauty has consequences.

Remove three weeks from your social calendar, four if you want to be absolutely sure no tell-tale bruising will still be evident. You'll look presentable in two weeks, better in three weeks and terrific in four weeks. It may take an additional week or two to get back to the same energy level that you had prior to your surgery.

There are several personal preparations that you can make prior to the surgery. If your "roots" are showing or if its time for your biannual bodywave, have them taken care of at least two weeks before surgery. Otherwise, the chemical process will leave your hair porous and it will tangle and snarl itself beneath your initial head dressing the first post-operative night. You don't want any caustic chemicals on your suture lines for at least six weeks after surgery, so no hair coloring or body waves during this time.

It's beneficial to have an exfoliating facial the day before surgery. This will deep-clean your pores and get rid of dead skin. Wash your hair thoroughly the night before surgery and don't apply any sprays. You may rinse with a mild conditioner to prevent snarling after surgery when your hair is under the head dressing. If your surgeon has given you a sleeping pill to take the night before surgery, it is important to take it.

Plan to arrive at your surgeon's office with at least ten minutes to spare on the day of your surgery. You do not want to arrive stressed for fear of being late. Do not wear make-up or jewelry. This is no time for vanity and "glitz" has no place in the operating room. I remember an incident where a 1+ carat diamond earring came off with the patient's disposable O.R. cap after surgery. It was later located in the surgical trash. It would place the surgeon's staff in a very embarrassing position should an article of jewelry come up missing. Jewelry is also a hazard to the patient if electrical cauterizing equipment is used.

Wear something loose fitting, easy to put on and take off. A sweat suit with a zip-front is appropriate. Bring a small light-weight duffel bag or suitcase that your personal belongings can be placed in during your surgery. Warm socks sometimes come in handy in the recovery room should you feel cold. A large head scarf makes your departure from the office a little less conspicuous.

You will leave surgery with a pressure head dressing and perhaps two drains assuring good flap adhesion (50% of cosmetic surgeons do not use drains, only a tight dressing). A certain amount of swelling and bruising will be evident at this time and can continue to increase for twenty-four to forty-eight hours. Remember, the sides of our bodies differ, therefore, it may be necessary to perform more extensive surgery on one side of your face than on the other to maintain symmetry in the final results. This may cause more swelling and bruising on one side than on the other.

Any sharp pain, particularly if it is not relieved by your pain medication, should be reported immediately to your surgeon. Generally, there is only slight discomfort, a feeling of pulling or pressure which is relieved with a prescribed pain medication.

Although it is not a common occurrence, and can happen no matter who the surgeon may have been, there is a complication referred to as a "hematoma". When this complication occurs, pain/swelling and discoloration are the presenting symptoms at the surgical site. The cause is a blood vessel or vessels that may start bleeding after surgery has been completed and if not diagnosed, could cause sloughing or permanent damage to the surface skin due to a jeopardized blood supply. If detected early, this fluid can be aspirated with a syringe and needle. It may be necessary to return to surgery so the flap of skin under which the fluid is collected can be drained, the leaking vessel repaired, and a new pressure dressing applied. It may mean an extra week involved in the healing process due to the additional bruising, but the final cosmetic results are usually not affected.

A good rule is not to concentrate on a mirror for at least seven days postoperatively. By then the swelling has begun to diminish and the bruising is now at the yellow-green stage versus the red-purple. If your surgeon permits, you can begin applying warm towels to the remaining bruised areas of your neck after the fourth to fifth day. This will increase the blood flow to the area and assist in washing away the dead blood cells that are causing the discoloration.

For the first ten nights you should lay with your head elevated on several pillows to assist gravity with the run-off of the swelling. For the first forty-eight hours lay with your chin elevated, staring at the ceiling, so good circulation can reestablish itself beneath your chin. This is because, more than likely, your surgeon liposuctioned some of the excess fat from beneath your chin, and tied up the muscle structure to prevent sagging in the future. You should also be looking straight forward and not to the left or right. Maintain this position when sleeping at night. Turning your head to one side or the other will result in gravity assisting the swelling to drain to the lower side.

You may experience some discomfort during the first three days. Don't be a martyr, take your pain medication as prescribed. Pain causes an elevation in vital signs. When your blood pressure increases, more stress is placed on the hundreds of tiny capillaries that are rebuilding themselves to establish new collateral circulation. Some of them may break causing additional bruising.

Keep the talking to a minimum the first forty-eight hours, the movement of the mandible (lower jaw) has the same effect as an increased blood pressure. It physically abuses the small capillaries and you end up with the same results, more bruising.

Your diet the first night should be clear fluids. The next day you can start on your soft diet which should continue for forty-eight hours. A soft diet can include mashed potatoes, soups, eggs, pureed vegetables, puddings, ice cream, yogurt, smoothies, etc. Then progress to chopped, mashed, and diced food so that no major chewing is required for at least a week. Do not put hot liquids or food in your mouth, let them cool to lukewarm. Heat will draw blood to the area and this would only put added pressure on your small blood vessels.

As mentioned, you will look good in two weeks, better in three, and terrific in four. By the end of the thirtieth day your bruising should be completely healed and the outward signs of your surgery should be gone, with the exception of pink suture lines tucked into your hairline and behind your ears. These can be hidden with minor efforts on the part of your hairdresser or yourself.

Remember, you have had anesthesia, a small amount of blood loss, and surgery, so your energy level may take four to six weeks to get back to where it was pre-operatively. Be patient, baby yourself a little, and the new beautiful woman will slowly reveal herself. You can start exercising between the fourth and sixth week depending on your doctor's preference and the extent of your surgical procedures.

During the initial seven days after surgery it is important to continue good suture care. Use a Q-tip to apply hydrogen peroxide two to three times a day to your suture lines once your surgeon has removed your head dressing and given his approval. He may also have you apply an antibiotic ointment to your suture lines for the first week post-operatively or until all of your sutures have been removed. The peroxide will keep your suture lines clean, assist in preventing infection, and promote healing. "Blue Ice" packs found in the First Aid section of your pharmacy are also an added source of comfort when cooled in the freezer, wrapped in a napkin or linen towel, and placed along side your cheeks two or three times a day. The coolness feels soothing and assists with reducing the swelling.

It is also important to remember not to get in a "head-down" position which would increase the blood flow to the head. Let someone else look under the bed for the missing slipper. When getting out of bed, sit on the edge of the bed for fifteen seconds before standing, make certain your head is clear and you do not feel weak. Once this is established, stand by the bed for another five seconds to make certain that you will continue to feel strong and not light-headed. You do not want to become faint and risk a fall. This applies primarily to your first forty-eight hours after surgery. It's important to remember not to use hot blow dryers or curling irons near your scalp after surgery.

Your surgeon will tell you when you can once again get behind the wheel of a car. Although you may feel strong enough to drive I want to point out a very important fact. Should you have the misfortune of getting into an automobile accident that inflicts injury on someone else, your liability would be greatly increased. It is a known fact that bruising and swelling of the neck area prohibits rapid movement of the head for good side to side visual assessment. Your defense would be very weak.

A facelift is one of the finest presents a woman can bestow upon herself. I remember the woman who, unbeknownst to her husband, withdrew $30,000.00 from their savings account to pay for a facelift by a Beverly Hills surgeon. She had rationalized that his alcoholic intake and cigarette consumption over the twenty years they had been married had surpassed this amount. She took pleasure in every penny spent, and not even his wrath upon discovery tainted her joy in her new appearance.

Many times women will undergo their surgery without informing their spouses who were usually away on a business trip at the time. I did feel, however, that the woman who had undergone a facelift, breast implants, and a tummy tuck without informing her husband, and still did not expect him to notice, was being a bit unrealistic.

Chin Implant

(MENTOPLASTY)

There are several reasons to consider a chin augmentation or "chin implant". Obviously a weak, small chin comes to mind first. However, as you age, your skin sags around the chin area. Your surgeon may elect to insert a chin implant to assist in adding longevity to your facelift as an implant offers a supportive substructure.

There's always the possibility you've had a weak profile all your life but elected to ignore it, or perhaps it didn't bother you. Now is an excellent time to address it. It is a very simple procedure when in combination with a facelift and even when done as a single procedure.

Your surgeon has a multitude of shapes and sizes to choose from. He may even insert different implants during surgery to actually visualize which one is the most complimentary to your facial structure.

The actual insertion site is most often through the mouth. A one and a half to two inch incision is made at the base of your lower lip and gum. Dissolvable sutures are then used to close the incision leaving no external evidence of surgery.

Post-operatively you'll experience discomfort for three to four days due to swelling. A supportive external taping is applied to the chin to help reduce this swelling and hold the implant in place. As with any implant, it's advisable to be placed on an antibiotic for four to five days post-operatively to prevent infection. The swelling subsides 50% within the first week with the rest reducing gradually over a two to three week period. A chin implant greatly enhances your facial profile both from a side and frontal view.

If a chin implant is elected due to a weak, or non-existing chin, it can be done in the late teens. Although the chin bone continues to grow into the early twenties, an implant can effectively be inserted earlier, and will stay in proportion through future growth if properly sized when inserted. It can make a big difference in a teenager's self-esteem by greatly improving their appearance.

Cheek Implants

One of the latest innovations on the part of the beauty makers (implant manufacturers) is the cheek implant. Made of Silicone and anatomically contoured for the three distinct areas of the cheeks most often needing improvement, the implant is placed in either the infra-orbital sill, the lateral orbital rim, or mid-facial area, offering width to the face. This is where the artistic talents of your surgeon take over as he molds your new image in his mind, and then creates it on his surgical table. The placement of the implants can determine a deeper set eye and more prominent and feminine profile.

The insertion site is through your mouth. A small incision is made between your upper lip and gum. It is virtually painless post-operatively but the ensuing swelling of the cheek can cause discomfort for a few days. You will lose your ability to smile until the swelling dissipates in five to seven days. You should rinse your mouth with hydrogen peroxide after eating to keep the incision site clean. Cold compresses to your cheeks post-operatively help minimize swelling and bruising.

Cheek implants offer a subtle enhancement to your facial profile. Virtually undetectable, they offer a mysterious visual presentation, keeping the admirer guessing as to just what has taken place to make you look so good.

Chemical Peel

Now that we have the face relocated to its original position, let's address the skin. The extent of skin damage, as previously stated, depends on the amount of time spent in the sun, your smoking addiction, and genetic make-up. Weather is another enemy, cold winds and temperatures can also play havoc on your complexion. Some women have very large unsightly pores. Large pores, leathery sun damaged skin, wrinkles, and the crepe-like skin, and tiny little lines that appear around the eyes, are all good reasons to seek a chemical peel.

A chemical peel smoothes out your skin by chemically removing the outer layer (or layers depending on the strength of the peel) of your skin. Small wrinkles and lines also disappear.

The beautifying results of a peel are usually long lasting, but it does not prevent new aging from taking place in five to fifteen years. The length of time depends, once again, on your sun exposure and smoking habits.

Women in their forties very often get a peri-oral peel. This peel is just around the mouth for fine vertical lines that begin to form outward from the lips. A peri-orbital peel is just around the eyes. It helps to minimize the tiny lines and wrinkles that creep in undetected and can even assist somewhat with the creping condition that is so unsightly. A full face peel may not be necessary until your fifties or sixties.

A full face peel can be done six weeks after a facelift. The surgeon will first determine whether or not your skin tone is conducive to a peel. Orientals and dark-skinned women do not make good candidates, as a peel may exhibit a lighter pigmented line between peeled and non-peeled skin.

It's important to note that there are two chemicals available for use. The first is TCA or Trichloracetate. This is used for your light peels and has minimal side effects. The second is Phenol, generally used when a deep peel is necessary. Women with histories of heart disease should be aware that Phenol is absorbed into the blood stream and can irritate the heart. This is generally not a problem to the healthy person, but to a woman with a history of arrhythmias or cardiac disorders it could prove a problem.

You are sedated lightly while the chemical is applied slowly and in layers. It is applied with cotton swabs and a layer of tape is sometimes applied over the entire face. Swelling will start immediately and a burning sensation occurs for twenty-four to forty-eight hours, pain medication is available.

Rest in bed with your head elevated to assist gravity with the run-off of the swelling. Sometimes a fan in the room stirs up the air and assists with relieving some of the burning. Your surgeon may also recommend the application of cold through wet or dry methods depending on the presence of tape. The swelling may take seven to ten days to subside. The tape is usually removed on the third day. Take a pain pill forty-five minutes prior to your doctor's appointment as this can be a painful procedure. Your new, vital skin will remain pink for two weeks and slowly fade for the next six.

It is easy to allow yourself to become depressed during your first week of recuperation. Cover your mirrors if this helps. Don't forget that the butterfly was first an unattractive worm, although I'm not sure that thought will offer much consolation, just remember, "This too shall pass."

The Aging Nose

This will come as a surprise to many women, but as you age, your nose begins to droop. If you think of it logically it makes perfect sense. As your complete face begins to lose its elasticity and sag, so goes the nose, especially the tip. A nasal tip that begins to fall, since it is the mid focal point of the face, gives the entire face a fallen or droopy expression. A nasal tip elevation gives a more youthful appearance.

Throughout life, you may have banged your nose accidentally, and didn't realize that inner damage was sustained. Breathing may have been impaired, but not enough to warrant a trip to the doctor. You adjusted to your restricted breathing, and soon forgot the pleasure of the added breathing of open air passages. It is possible you may have damaged your septum which can be repaired by a Rhinoplasty at the same time that the nasal tip is raised.

If you have lived your life with a bulbous tip or a hump on the bridge of your nose, you may consider corrective surgery at this time. Make certain that if you elect to undergo a Rhinoplasty that you have all desired revisions completed at one time.

There are several reasons why a Rhinoplasty is not a pleasurable surgery. Swelling will take place after surgery resulting in an inability to breath through your nasal passages.

Mouth breathing is then necessary causing dry lips and mouth. Vaseline gauze is very often used to pack your nostrils after surgery. This is to maintain your new inner structure and provide pressure which will control bleeding. Packing is removed from the second to the fourth day. A nasal cast or taping is often placed over the exterior bridge of the nose to maintain placement of the rearranged cartilage. It also protects it from accidental exterior blows. The cast or taping may be left on from five to seven days.

Post-operatively, it is comforting to have lemon/glycerin swabs available to wipe out and refresh the mouth. A small amount of blood may have been swallowed during surgery causing nausea and vomiting at this time. Should you vomit this old blood do not be concerned as it will relieve the nausea. Should bleeding and vomiting persist contact your surgeon. Your nose may continue to drip for a few days, taping a small gauze in place under your nostrils to absorb this minimizes the inconvenience. You may even experience the need to blow your nose at intervals for several months after surgery. Using a Q-tip, place a small amount of Vaseline just inside each nostril to help prevent uncomfortable crusting from forming. Placing a small amount of mentholated ointment, such as Vicks, on your upper lip, offers vapors that help keep nasal passages open.

Some surgeons suggest squirting a saline spray into the nostrils for added moisture. It is important not to insert any object into the nostril, only to the opening.

Because the nose is one of the least vascular areas of the body and also protrudes in a manner that makes gravity a difficult method of relieving swelling, it may take six to ten months to actually shrink down to its intended size.

After the tenth day of your surgery, when your packing has been removed for several days, you may feel more comfortable if you thinly coat the lining of the nostrils with a small amount of Vaseline on a Q-tip at bedtime. This will facilitate easier breathing and prevent crust or hardened secretions from forming. Your saline spray can still be used during the day.

The discomforts I have described are more inconveniences than painful. The final results far supersede the post-operative discomfort... open air passages, straightened bridge, raised tip, refined nose. The choices are yours.

Breast Augmentation

Breast augmentation is just another name for breast implants. Breast implant surgery knows no age boundary. The forty year old woman who has been flat-chested all her life may decide its time to see what it's like to fill out a "C" cup. The twenty year old wants to take advantage of this modern surgical technology to further enhance her body, increase her cleavage, and attract men. We also have the woman who has breast fed her children, and is left with flat drooping breasts due to her now missing under-carriage. Then again, we have the thirty-five to forty-five year old woman whose husband has just left her for a younger more curvaceous female, and the desire to excel in the areas of personal body image takes over. She diets, becomes a member of a gym, buys new more revealing clothes, undergoes liposuction, enhances the color of her hair, gets her teeth whitened, has acrylic nails applied, and augments her breasts.

There are numerous reasons why a woman may elect to undergo breast implants, but whatever the reason, once the decision has been made, there is no changing her mind.

Until 1992 the number of breast implant surgeries increased yearly. There are now millions of women who have undergone breast augmentation. This really is no wonder in a world where a growing emphasis is placed on sexuality and sensuality in every phase of media and entertainment. Whether right or not, a woman's self esteem is increased, and her feeling of sexuality is doubled, as a result of breast implants.

Women also note an increased feeling of femininity and desirability after implant surgery. Very few women will part with their implants once inserted.

The controversy surrounding silicone gel implants and consequential health problems relates to the possible rupturing of the implant. Some studies indicate that this results in the leakage of silicone gel into the surrounding autoimmune system. A study in 2010 by the ASPS showed 296, 203 breast augmentations and 93, 083 breast reconstructions used 50/50 gel and saline implants. Although better than no implants at all, saline implants do have a tendency to give a less than satisfactory shape to the breast and have been known to have a slight "sloshing" sound upon movement. They are not an acceptable alternative to gel implants but are an interim solution until research rules on the safety of the gel implant. Hopefully, a satisfactory substitute will be developed that will contain a substance that will be harmlessly reabsorbed by the body should an implant rupture or leak. The F.D.A. is now allowing Board Certified Plastic Surgeons to insert silicone gel implants once again. Make your own informed decision as to which type is best for you.

Breast augmentation surgery takes 1 ½ to 3 hours depending on whether the implant is under or over the muscle and is done under general anesthesia. The incision site should be the decision of both surgeon and patient. Three sites are possible and the incision is usually 1 to 1.5 inches in length. Some surgeons prefer to locate the incision in the areola of the nipple, either straight across the areola or around the outer lower edge of the nipple. This offers asymmetry in scar location and is visually more confusing to detect. However, a nipple incision means scar tissue formation in an area of a woman's body where sensation can be affected by its presence. As most women know, this is not an area where sensation is readily parted with. The second choice is the lower fold of the breast. This area does not interfere with sensation but is visible when the woman lies on her back or her breast is lifted. In this location, the under-support seams/elastic/wire of a bra can cause pressure and irritation resulting in discomfort. The third alternative is the axillary approach. A one inch incision is made in the axilla (armpit) which fades with time and in no way interferes with the natural appearance of the breast, an ideal solution. However, verify that your surgeon is adept at this procedure as it does entail a more distant approach over the rib carriage and additional skill.

There is also a choice in the actual placement of the implant itself. It can be placed between the breast tissue and the muscle covering the chest wall, or between the muscle and the chest wall. Here again, the woman should have full knowledge of this placement. There is slightly less incidence of encapsulation with the implant between the muscle and the chest wall, and it is less likely to interfere with breast feeding should the woman be of child-bearing age. However, the surgery is more painful during the first four days of the recovery period and the breast will have a tendency to be less free-moving due to the overlaying muscle structure. This will relax with time.

Locating the implant between the breast tissue and the muscle wall is less painful as the creation of the capsule to hold the implant does not involve the undermining of any muscle tissue. It does, however, have an increased incidence of the formation of scar tissue which can make the implant become firm and painful requiring replacement. There is also the possibility that the formation of scar tissue could interfere with breast feeding as breast tissue is involved. Breast infections when breast feeding may also become more prevalent when the implant is in this location.

It is important to discuss the size of the implant with your surgeon. Make certain that you both visualize the same size breast as an end result. Ask to see the implant that he plans to insert. Implants come in several sizes and shapes and this simple request can avoid a post-operative disappointment for a breast size that is either too small or too large. Make note of the manufacturer of your implant and its exact content, it's your body, know what goes into it.

Many women do not realize that a "capsule" must be created for the retention of the implant. A capsule is the undermining of the tissue to create an envelope, or sac, in which the implant can move freely about. The sac usually extends from one inch below the clavicle to within 3/4" of the sternum, and to the midline under the axilla. The floor of the sac remains the same as the existing breast. This sac allows the implant to move normally with different body positioning, an important factor especially when lying on your back. When in this position the normal breast falls to the side, it does not remain perched on top of your chest and neither should your implants.

If this sac should close, or encapsulate, due to the formation of scar tissue, the implant becomes hard and fixed in one location, becoming unnatural in appearance and painful for the woman. Surgery is required to correct this condition. Some surgeons will try to "pop" the sac open again by applying external pressure to the breast or squeezing it between their palms using every ounce of their strength. This is an extremely painful procedure and offers only temporary relief to the problem, should it help at all. I advise against it. That much pressure to any human tissue can not be beneficial and, without doubt, could rupture an implant.

No one knows the cause of the formation of scar tissue. Different types of implants have been designed to prevent its occurrence but have not been 100% successful.

After your breast implant surgery a pressure dressing is applied through the use of ace bandages or stretch surgical tape. It is not uncommon for a surgeon to insert drains to assist in draining off fluid that can form during the healing process. This drain may be removed within one to three days post-operatively. Pain is present due to the creation of the capsule and the stretching of the breast to accommodate the implant. This pain is relieved with prescribed medication for the first three to four days. Post-operatively, it is important to rest with the chest elevated on several pillows to facilitate the drainage of fluids and prevent swelling. Elbows should be kept at your sides for the first two to three days, followed by restricted activity for one week. Do not lift more than two pounds for up to ten days. A week of rest should be allotted for. Sutures are removed in four to six days. The incisions can be kept clean during the healing period by cleansing them with hydrogen peroxide and applying an antibiotic ointment.

Underwire bras should not be worn, the wire can cause a crimp in the implant if not positioned properly and this can not be corrected. Many surgeons recommend wearing no bra at all, only camisoles. They feel the free movement of the implant within the breast allows the implant to move fully about the capsule and diminishes the formation of scar tissue, a viable thought.

If breast augmentation is not successful it can be very traumatizing emotionally. Sometimes the body continually rejects the implant through constant encapsulation, the woman must then have the implants permanently removed. This would return her to her smaller breast size, a breast that now exhibits even more drooping due to the stretching that occurred to accommodate the implant. This possibility should be taken into consideration prior to a woman's final decision to have the surgery.

Breast Reduction With or Without Augmentation

(MASTOPEXY)

By the time you have reached your forties, gravity has generally played a major role in the location of your nipple line. Once located approximately three to four inches below your armpit and pointing straight ahead, it now measures six to eight inches below your armpit and may even be pointing directly at the floor. Its once sexual attraction has taken back seat to comical relief. There is an answer, and it's called a Mastopexy with Augmentation if necessary. This translates to a breast reduction with the use of an implant to offer a new foundation.

There are usually two suture lines in the shape of an inverted "T". The first starts at the nipple line and goes straight down to the second which follows the normal contour of the lower breast. It does require relocating the nipple so there will be a minute suture line around the areolar or outer rim of the nipple. It is important to note that loss of sensation in the nipple is an end result, so you should take this into consideration when contemplating this surgery.

Post-operatively, you'll find yourself in a tightly wrapped bandage around your chest area. Pressure from the bandage maintains good suture line approximation and prevents bleeding. You may have a drain in for two to three days to draw off any fluid that may be produced during the healing process.

Once again you should lay with your shoulders elevated on pillows to assist gravity with reducing the swelling that takes place during the healing process. Your elbows should be kept at your sides, do not raise your arms in an upward motion. This is to prevent stress on suture lines or misplacement of the implant. Immobilization for two to three days reduces risk of complications. Needless to say you do not lift anything at all for the first forty-eight hours, and nothing over two pounds for the next ten days.

There is discomfort involved that is relieved by medication. By the fourth day you are feeling much improved as the drains have generally been removed and the swelling has started to subside. Ice packs the first two to three days offer comfort and reduce swelling. Place them on your upper chest and under your armpits. When the dressings are removed you will be placed in a stretch fabric bra for good support.

It is extremely important to observe that a blood supply is maintained to the transplanted nipples. Their color should remain pink. If any dark areas develop in the color of the areolar, call your doctor immediately.

Breast reductions are not only done in the over-forty set, teenagers with oversized breasts are also seeking this procedure. Having it performed in their youth will save stress on their spinal column and heckling in the arena of life.

Tummy Tuck

(ABDOMINOPLASTY)

A woman doesn't usually place much emphasis on her flat stomach during her youth. She takes it for granted until she becomes pregnant and then it becomes the focal point of her life. She watches and admires as it becomes rounder and rounder. Protruding out beyond her toes, growing and growing. Perhaps she rubs baby oil on it nightly to help prevent stretch marks, perhaps she's never heard of such a practice and then again she may have never heard about stretch marks. Skin tone (elasticity) is genetic, as previously stated, some women have never experienced a stretch mark and never will.

Pregnancy stretches not only the skin but the underlying muscle structure. Each pregnancy causes additional weakness and damage. It becomes harder and harder to get back into shape after delivery. The St. John knits are now in the back of the closet where the V-neck dresses used to be. There's nothing worse than a knit full of belly.

Even without childbearing, women have a tendency to develop a "pooch" (bulging fatty area) in their lower abdominal wall. Not very sexy to say the least. It can cause their panties to roll downward and their belts to ride upward.

There is an answer, have that belly surgically excised by a procedure known as an Abdominoplasty, (taking a tuck out of the tummy).

The exact purpose of this surgery is to remove as much excess skin and fat as possible and tighten up the underlying muscle structure. The only catch is that the navel must be repositioned or it will find itself relocated somewhere between your hip bones. Abdominoplasty only removes the stretch marks that are located directly on the excess skin that is removed. The result of this surgery is a flat, or flatter, abdomen. Yes, you will still be able to bend over, no, it will not cinch your waist or reduce your buttock area. The good news is that it is generally permanent, however, the tightened muscles can loosen again.

It is best to have this surgery when pregnancy is no longer a factor in your life. Excessive new weight gain will, of course, be evidenced in this area.

An abdominoplasty is considered major surgery and is performed under general anesthesia. It is important to note that the incision line is quite long. The horizontal incision runs from iliac crest (hipbone) to iliac crest, dipping downward through the pubic hair line. It does fade and flatten with time.

If your tummy needs major alterations, it may mean four days of discomfort post-operatively. The recovery period involves a week of very limited activity. It includes bedrest in a jack-knife (shoulders elevated, knees flexed) position for two days, with bathroom and chair privileges only. Your immediate post-operative care may include some intravenous fluids for twenty-four to forty-eight hours. An abdominal drain may be inserted during surgery and left in place for two to three days. You will be allowed limited walking in a bent-over position for the next two days, and an additional week of pampering and continued limited activity should be adhered to.

No lifting for three weeks and then with moderation. You will feel "tight" for two to three weeks. Your energy may not reach its pre-surgical level for five to six weeks, but you can usually return to work in three weeks depending on your job.

It is best to wear a good abdominal support garment for four to six weeks. Abdominal swelling may make your waistline thicker for a few weeks after surgery, but the swelling will subside. The support garment will help hold the tummy in and the added support will feel good.

Thighs, and Buttocks Lift

Why stop now! We're just starting to get surgically creative. Now that the tummy is nipped and tucked why should we be content with convoluted thighs and fannies. I must warn you, if your knees are also layered, this surgery will not alter them. There is a limit to the capability of cosmetic surgery.

If weight problems added to your present state, be sure that your weight has now stabilized, and you have lost as much as you intend to.

General anesthesia is indicated and the surgery may take two to three hours. The incision for the thigh lift is a semi-circle located in your natural lap fold between leg and abdomen. The skin is lifted with some undermining required, excess fat removed, and the extra skin cut out. Edges are approximated, sutured, and a drain is sometimes inserted for two to three days. A surgical dressing and support garment is then put in place.

The buttocks lift can be done at the same time or separately. The same basic procedure is repeated, but it does not require the undermining of skin, as the convoluted fanny folds are more localized and accessible. The incision is located slightly high on the buttock. This is because time and gravity will soon lower it to the natural fold of the leg-buttock crease. Your surgeon will remove excess fat beneath the skin, cut off the excess skin, and suture the approximated edges. Once again, a drain may be inserted, and a dressing and support garment put in place.

There will be pain at the surgical sites for two to three days, medication will be ordered. The discomfort will lessen each day, up to the seventh day post-op. Your legs will swell after this surgery and you will need to wear support stockings for at least two weeks. Make sure that you give yourself a full two weeks for recuperation with a third week optional as you do not want to rush your recovery. You will be allowed to shower after the drains have been removed, usually the third day. Do not sit in a tub of water as you do not want bath water to seep into your incisions.

Scars are a factor to take into consideration with these operations. Although partially obscured in natural folds they may widen with time, especially if enough quiet-time is not allowed post-operatively for proper healing. Sex is taboo for at least three weeks post-operatively, and then only after your surgeon's OK.

If you have a medical history of phlebitis, the abdominoplasty and thigh and buttocks lift surgeries may be contraindicated. Consult with your medical doctor.

Arm Lift

(BRACHIOPLASTY)

If you have either experienced excessive weight loss, or the passage of the years have given way to "upper arm flab", there is a surgical procedure available. The Arm Lift may not incite the urge to fully expose your arms again, but it will present a more proportioned body image and perhaps help your clothes fit better. Suture lines are visible as they are placed beneath your arm. The surgery removes excess skin. It can return in time, but it would take many years before more surgery was needed.

The cause of this loose skin is usually due to the diminishing of underlying muscle tone. If you work out a lot and then stop, you may see this loose skin as a result. Excessive weight loss and the general passage of years are contributing factors.

The surgery takes place under intravenously administered anesthesia. The incision may extend from the armpit to the elbow depending on the amount of excess skin. It is placed in the under-arm area. Excess skin and underlying fat will be removed.

Your arms will swell and ache, you will require pain medication for one to two days. Keep your arms elevated on pillows to assist with the run-off of the swelling by giving gravity an added advantage. Bruising and swelling may be evidenced for two weeks.

You can usually return to work in a week but NO lifting until your surgeon approves. Your arms may ache more readily for two to three weeks. No sex for two weeks as you do not want to experience inadvertent arm movements.

Liposuction

Popularized in the Eighties, Liposuction is one of our fastest growing procedures. The correct term is Suction Assisted Lipectomy (SAL), or suctioning of the fat.

Women have been trying to look slimmer for centuries through the use of corsets, diets, dark colored clothing, simple straight-line clothing styles etc. etc. Now we're having fat sucked out of our bodies through surgical methods. Some say we're crazy, others just enjoy their new size eight. Knees and ankles that were once chubby can now be slim. Saddlebag, or thunder-thighs, can be reduced, chubby-cheeks can now be hollowed, and most areas of the body can be "sculptured" or fine-tuned to a slimmer you.

It sounds like magic, but it is serious surgery. SAL is done by inserting a cannula, a long metal instrument connected to a strong vacuum/suction machine, into the fat layers of the body. Fat cells are sucked out but it also takes with it a certain amount of blood and body fluids. Most surgeons will not remove more than the equivalent of eight to nine pounds of body weight. More than that and you're tempting to imbalance the body's ability to readjust.

There is pain and a certain amount of risk involved. The surgery is done under general anesthesia and the length of time it takes depends on the number of areas to be suctioned. If your surgeon is not experienced in the procedure, it is possible to perforate a major blood vessel or organ, and incur hemorrhage/infection/death. If the cannula is not guided skillfully, it can enter muscle or body organs and inflict tears and additional pain.

If a surgeon is planning on removing in excess of four to five pounds of body fat, he may request that you contribute one to two units of your own blood in the weeks previous to your surgery. This is to insure adequate fluid replacement after surgery, with minimal risk from blood contamination, by transfusing you with your own blood post-operatively.

You will leave the operating room in a stretch garment specifically designed for liposuction patients. Depending upon the areas suctioned, the garment may reach from your waist to your ankles.

You should plan on at least three days of intermittent bedrest. Many doctors will state that the discomfort is equivalent to feeling "lame" after heavy exercising. I equivocate it to being hit by a Mack truck. If eight to nine pounds have been extracted from abdomen, thighs, and hips, you will be in pain for twenty-four to forty-eight hours. Pain medication is prescribed. Rest in bed with your knees flexed to relax the abdominal muscles. If not in an electric bed place a pillow under your knees and keep your shoulders elevated. Attack the problem from both ends. Ambulation is very important to healing. Ambulate 3-4 times a day, even if painful.

You'll love the liposuction body girdle. It extends from the waist to the knees, fastens on each side of the body with hooks and eyes supplementing a full length zipper. It should be worn for a full two weeks, night and day. It is designed with an open crotch area, for those personal moments, so it is very important that it is properly aligned when zipped in place. A three to four inch funnel placed strategically inside the parameters of the crotch opening facilitates urination without getting your lipogirdle wet and consequently stained and odorous. I suggest leaving the doctor's office with two girdles, so one can be in the wash while the other is on the body. They cost $100 - $200 depending on size.

The girdle offers compression to the areas liposuctioned to help prevent swelling and bruising, thus minimizing the discoloration. It also assists in reminding the skin it must shrink a small amount to adhere to the underlying tissue. I mention the reference to prevention of bruising with tongue-in-cheek, as there is extensive bruising with this procedure. One does not have a four to six inch cannula thrust in and out of their body forty to fifty times without incurring bruising. This bruising takes three to four weeks to disappear.

Small ridges may be felt under the skin where the cannula "tracked". You can help these ridges smooth over by soaping your hands each time you shower or take a bath, and rubbing the liposuctioned areas in a circular motion, use only light pressure. No hot or steamy showers or baths for seven to ten days after surgery, only warm.

Plan on a full week for recuperation if large areas are involved. After the third day you will recuperate at a faster rate than the first three due to the swelling and discomfort. It is very important that you drink a lot of liquids after surgery to help the body replace the water it lost in the fat removed. Drinking liquids will not make you gain weight or swell more excessively, it will help balance your body fluids.

The results of liposuction can be permanent if a proper diet and exercise program is followed. Remember, liposuction is not a substitute for diet, and should not be used as a means to "lose weight". Liposuction is to remove excess fat from specific areas of the body where you have not been successful in reducing through diet or exercise. In a woman, these areas are most often her abdomen and hips.

Most people who undergo liposuction are very pleased with their results within thirty days. Sometimes the results are quite dramatic, resulting in the need for a new wardrobe. Tsk, tsk.

Filling in and Plumping Out

At this point I know you may have figured out where your nasal-labial folds are, but I'm certain you never knew you had a glabella. Your nasal-labial folds are the creases extending from the corner of your nostrils to the outer edges of your lips. Your glabella is the area between your eyebrows, also known as your "frown lies". They become more prominent with the passage of years. Squinting and frowning accentuate the glabella lines. Ironically, smiling and laughter accentuate the nasal-labial lines. Who said, "Laughter is the best medicine"?

Fillers are used to plump up lips, fill in lines between the eyebrows, flatten out wrinkles around the eyes and mouth, or even fill indented scars or pock marks. They used to use silicone and collagen extensively but silicone travels and can't be relied upon to stay where it is injected. Many people are allergic to Collagen, so neither were the perfect solution. Your own fat harvested from another part of your body can also be used, but it is not always convenient.

Hyaluronic Acid based fillers have been approved by the F.D.A.. This is a substance found in all cells and the belief is that no one is allergic to this product. It is found in many fillers: Captique, Perlane, Elevess, Juvaderm, Cosmo Derm (Inamed), Hylaform, Restylane, Zyplast. It is believed that Restylane lasts longest for deeper applications. Results last from five to six months.

Lips have a tendency to shrink with the aging process. They lose natural collagen making them thin. There are also women who were either born with a thin lip line or just want a plumper, pouty look to their lips. This is now possible.

Injecting lips can be quite painful and requires a dental block when done as a separate procedure. If done at the same time as a facelift it is quite common, and permanent, to have the severed tissue threaded into the lips. The body will not reject it's own tissue and it will not be reabsorbed. Discuss it with your surgeon.

Treat post-injection areas with ice compresses to reduce swelling. This will subside in a few days. It is always smart to consider the injection of fillers in conjunction when planning surgical procedures that require anesthesia.

Multiple Procedures

You may be wondering just how many procedures you can safely undergo at one time. No one likes to go under anesthesia more often than necessary.

If you are in good general health and have a sound medical history, 6.5 hours of sedation is a reasonable length of time to consider. Most women are interested in more than one cosmetic procedure to be performed at one given time. Improvements in surgical techniques and anesthesia make multiple procedures more commonplace and with fewer risks to the patient. The surgeon is responsible for determining his patient's medical candidacy for multiple procedures. It is also important for the patient to determine the surgeon's ability to endure a 6.5 hour procedure as it does take personal stamina. Request that your surgery be scheduled as the first to be performed that day. This will at least insure you of a 'fresh surgeon'.

Many women would prefer to recuperate from several procedures at one time, this limits the number of times they must remain out of their social circle. They prefer to "Get it all over with at once". They would rather endure the combined bandaging, swelling, bruising and discomfort post-operatively, and then emerge with a totally improved result.

There is also a cost benefit by undergoing multiple procedures. Most surgeons will reduce the cost of each procedure as the patient is already anesthetized and the surgical area prepared, this cuts down on his personal time involved. Strategically, it is a beneficial financial move for the surgeon to make as it will induce the patient to include more procedures, thus increasing the final cost.

Your surgeon should take into consideration the length of time it takes to complete each surgical procedure, and inform you of those that can be safely completed within the 6.5 hours of sedation. The following is a guideline to the time it generally takes to complete a procedure:

takes to complete a procedure:

Facelift	3 - 4 hrs.
Forehead/Brow Lift	1 -1.5 hrs.
Eyes (Upper & Lower Lids)	1 -1.5 hrs.
Rhinoplasty (Nose)	1 - 1.5 hrs.
Cheek Implants	45 - 60 min.
Chin Implant	30 min.
Breast Implants	1.5 - 2 hrs.
Breast Lift	2.5 - 3 hrs.
Breast Reduction	2.5 - 3 hrs.
Arm Lift	1.5 - 2 hrs.
Abdominoplasty (Tummy)	2.5 - 3.5 hrs
Liposuction (depending on areas)	1 - 3 hrs.
Buttocks Lift	2 - 2.5 hrs.
Thigh Lift	2 - 2.5 hrs.
Chemical Peel (full face)	1 - 1.5 hrs.

Section III

Surgeons That Excel

Surgeons That Excel

The surgeons in the following chapter are the true Masters of the nip and tuck. They are all located in the Beverly Hills area and are the famous "Surgeons to the Stars." I have based this list on 18 years of caring for their patients. This unique opportunity allowed me to assess and evaluate their patients based on the following:

1. *Amount of bruising and swelling*
2. *Amount of pain experienced*
3. *Amount of nausea*
4. *Number and type of complications*
5. *Placement of Suture Lines*
6. *Aesthetic surgical results*

I have indicated their certifications. Certification means that they have carried the seriousness of their profession to the highest level. Although complications from surgery and anesthesia cannot always be avoided, these surgeons have taken every precaution to see that their patients receive the finest in medical equipment and pre and post-operative care. Add the surgeon's skill to that combination and the surgical results can be only commendable.

I have emphasized the surgical procedures that each surgeon excels at. Not every surgeon performs every procedure with the same adeptness. It is important to choose a surgeon that excels in the procedures you desire.

In all fairness, there are other recovery retreats in Los Angeles and other surgeons that refer to them. My list does not represent every good surgeon in this town, only those whose work I have observed over the years.

It is important that you consult with at least three surgeons before selecting the one that you feel the most confidence in. Remember, you are entrusting him with your body and you only have one. You must trust him, respect him, and relate to him/her. Trepidation is a standard emotion when going under elective surgery, this can be kept at a minimum by the proper choice of your surgeon. They are listed alphabetically.

Dr. Gary Alter
416 North Bedford Dr., Suite 400
Beverly Hills, CA 90210
310 275 5566

Medical School:	UCLA School of Medicine
Residency:	Mayo Clinic, Rochester, Minnesota
Certifications:	American Board of Plastic Surgery
	American Board of Urology
Excels At:	Gender Reassignment (male to female, female to male) Penile Prosthesis, Penile Augmentation, Penile Reconstruction, Assessment of the sexually dysfunctional male. Facial Feminization, Breast Augmentation, Liposuction, Eyelid Surgery

Dr. Alter's professional expertise is plastic surgery of the male genitalia. His experience with gender reassignment surgery includes facial feminization, breast augmentation, and body sculpting. He is a skilled professional.

Dr. William Binder
120 S. Spalding Dr. Ste. 340
Beverly Hills, CA 90212
310 858 6749

Medical School:	New Jersey School of Medicine and Dentistry
Residency:	Mt. Sinai Hospital, New York City
Certified:	American Board of Facial Plastic and Reconstructive Surgery American Board of Otolaryngology
Excels At:	Facelifts, Cheek/Chin Implants, Botox, Rhinoplasty

Dr. Binder specializes in surgery of the head and neck. He received advanced training in Otolaryngology and head and neck surgery including facial plastic and reconstructive surgery while chief resident at Mount Sinai Hospital. Dr. Binder is one of the few doctors who has mastered the placement of facial implants, both chin and cheek. There is a definite art to this surgery as infection and other complications can occur.

Dr. Binder was one of the first surgeons to study the art of Botox placement in establishing maximum results in the treatment of facial wrinkles. He initiated the use of Botox for migraine headaches and published the first clinical research paper on the use of Botox for this purpose.

His office is modern and fully equipped. His operating room is state of the art and his staff professional and experienced. Your recovery room experience is detailed in advance to offer you the utmost in comfort and care.

Dr. Athleo Cambre
9201 West Sunset Blvd. Ste. 214
West Hollywood, CA 90069
310 777 6677

Medical School:	Case Western Reserve University, Cleveland, Ohio
Residency:	University of Colorado, Denver, Co. UCLA School of Medicine, L. A. CA
Diplomat:	American Board of Surgery
Diplomat:	American Board of Plastic Surgery
Specialty:	Facelift, Forehead, Eyelid Surgery, Breast Augmentation, Mastopexy, Abdominoplasty

Dr. Cambre's surgical prowess is worth expounding upon. He is meticulous in his surgical practice. His suture lines are perfectly approximated as he is dedicated to giving you the best results possible. He is able to perform equally well with face and body surgery so can complete a total makeover if desired.

I have watched his practice grow for the past ten years. I feel confident in referring him patients.

Dr. Alfred Cohen
414 N. Camden 8th Floor
Beverly Hills, CA 90210
310 275 5252

Medical School:	Tehran University School of Medicine
Residency:	Long Island Jewish-Hillside Medical Center
Certified:	American Board of Otolaryngology Head & Neck Surgery American Board of Facial Plastic and Reconstructive Surgery
Excels At:	Facial Surgery, Eyelid Surgery, Ear Surgery, Forehead Surgery

Dr. Cohen is a facelift surgeon. He has perfected his technique, his persona is strictly professional, and he is an extremely knowledgeable surgeon. He is a man of few words but skilled with a scalpel, and isn't that what we are seeking. He follows the course of his patient's recovery closely and does not like over medication as he feels it slows down the entire body's healing ability.

I remember a young seven year old boy who had a genetic ear protrusion. Although I did not see him pre-operatively, I understand from his mother that the condition was quite traumatic emotionally to the young child. They literally stuck out at a 45 degree angle from his head. Dr. Cohen pinned his ears, otoplasty, and the results changed the young man's life. The surgery is relatively simple in nature but has such a profound affect on a young person's enterplay with society.

Dr. Cohen shares the entire 8th floor of an office building with several associates. It's new, beautiful, and run by a staff of dedicated professionals. You are monitored throughout your anesthesia recovery by Registered Nurses and remain in the recovery room a minimum of 2 hours. This allows you to wake up, adjust to your post-operative condition (dressings, IV, foley) whatever the situation, and be discharged fully cognizant of your transfer.

Dr. Michael Groth
9675 Brighton Way Ste. 410
Beverly Hills, CA 90210
310 274 2525

Medical School: University of Miami, Fl.
Residency: UCLA, Jules Stein Institute, Los Angeles,
                    CA

Certified: American Board of Ophthalmology

Dr. Groth specializes in all surgeries to the eye including:

1. *Reconstruction of the eyelid*
2. *Correction of eyelid tumors*
3. *Use of Laser Blepharoplasty*
4. *Transconjunctival lower Blepharoplasty*
5. *Eyelid Lesion Reconstruction*
6. *Replacing fat to sunken lower lid*
7. *Aesthetic eyelid surgery*

Dr. Groth is the #1 go-to surgeon for surgery to the eye whether it be for eyelid rejuvenation, repair, or alteration, serious eye deformity, trauma, or disease.

Dr. Robert Hutcherson
9675 Brighton Way, Suite 410
Beverly Hills, CA 90210
310 276-7012

Medical School:	U.C.L.A. School of Medicine, CA
Residency:	General Surgery U.C.L.A.
	Head & Neck Surgery U.C.L.A.
Diplomate:	American Academy of Otolaryngology
Fellow:	American Academy of Facial Plastic and Reconstructive Surgery
Fellow:	American College of Surgeons
Fellow:	Society of Head and Neck Surgeons California Society of Facial Plastic Surgeons
Excels In:	Facelift, Endoscopic Forehead, Laser, Blepharoplasty

Dr. Hutcherson has my complete respect. He is one of the surgeons that quietly, and without fanfare, excels in professional expertise. He specializes in head and neck surgery, offering a deep plane facelift. His laser knowledge extends to the removal of port wine stains and the treatment of vascular malformations.

Dr. Lawrence Koplin
465 N. Roxbury, Ste 800
Beverly Hills, C A 90210
310 277 3223

Medical School:	Baylor College of Medicine, Houston, Tx.
Residency:	St. Joseph Hospital, Houston, Tx.
Certified:	American Board of Plastic Surgery
	American Board of Surgery
Excels At:	Facelifts, Eyelid Surgery, Rhinoplasty, Breast Surgery, Abdominoplasty, Liposuction

Dr. Koplin's life attitude is fully defined by his climbing Mount Kilimanjaro for his fiftieth birthday. He loves life's challenges and meets them head-on. He has the same zest for his profession.

Dr. Koplin is also an extreme makeover surgeon. His skills go from raising your forehead to sculpting your ankles. He is a full-service surgeon offering both facial and body rejuvenation. His tummy tucks are almost transparent, and his breast augmentations redefine bikinis. He is adept at liposuction and is fully in tune to proper body proportions.

From the custom designed, glass paneled entry doors to the hard wood floors and selected art, you know you are in the office of a professional.

Dr. Robert Kotler
9735 Wilshire Blvd. Suite 220
Beverly Hills, CA 90212
310 278 8721

Medical School:	Northwestern University, Chicago IL
Residency:	Cook County Hospital, Chicago, IL.
Diplomate:	American Board of Otolaryngology/Head and Neck Surgery
	American Board of Cosmetic Surgery
Excels At:	Permanent Non-Surgical Rhinoplasty, Rhinoplasty

I've had the privilege of caring for Dr. Kotler's patients for over fifteen years. He is at the very top of my list for nasal reconstruction, or rhinoplasty. Although he does exceptional facial surgery I have to admire his nose surgery and his facial peels.

Dr Kotler is the only surgeon I know that offers a deep phenol peel. Phenol is a strong acid that penetrates for serious sun damage or wrinkling. His results are phenomenal, it's like night to day. The recuperative time should be at least 30 days, although you will be through with the sloughing of the old skin by the 7th to 10th day. He applies tapes to the areas of skin in most distress and removes the tapes the second post-op day. This allows him to control the amount of acid treatment in the most damaged areas. There is a large amount of swelling with this procedure, but Dr. Kotler has his magic potions available that make the first ten post-operative days more comfortable.

Dr. Kotler is considered the Nose King of Beverly Hills. His experience with serious nose disfigurements, damage by previous nose surgerys, and reconstruction due to trauma, is extensive. Not many doctors will work on noses that have been previously surgically enhanced. Scarred or damaged cartilage is difficult and unpredictable.

Dr. Brent Moelleken
120 S. Spalding Ste. 110
Beverly Hills, CA 90212
310 273-1001

Medical School:	Yale University, School of Medicine
Residency:	University of California, San Francisco
Certified:	American Board of Plastic Surgery
Certified:	American Board of Surgery
Excels At:	Liposuction, Abdominoplasty, Facelift, Blepharoplasty, Breast Augmentation/ Reduction, Rhinoplasty, Coronal Surgery, Midface Lift

Dr. Moelleken's patient base is propelled by happy patients who literally expound on his surgical virtues. His surgeries are meticulously performed and his patients receive a very thorough post operative follow-through by him and his staff. He loves what he does and it is evident.

Dr. Moelleken is gifted in performing surgery both on the face and the body. He is especially adept at liposuction excelling in body sculpting. Liposuction is an art and should only be performed by skilled surgeons. Dr. Moelleken gained his reputation with SAL (Suction Assisted Lipectomy/sucking out of fat) ten years ago when word of his talents spread from satisfied patient to satisfied patient.

He takes his profession very seriously. Ego is not a word in his vocabulary which makes him especially endearing to me. His smile warms my heart every time I see him. His office is new with a private, adjoining, surgical suite. His staff is experienced, and knowledgeable. You are never alone in the recovery room which is a very important factor when choosing a surgeon.

When performing a facelift his protocol calls for removing your Jackson Pratt drains the following morning and reapplying a light head dressing. You may shampoo on the third post-operative day.

Dr. Moelleken is married to Dana Devon of Extra, between the two of them their social circles abound. She's a very lucky lady to have such a true gentleman in her life.

Dr. Leslie Stevens
201 S. Lasky Drive
Beverly Hills, CA 90212
310 556-1003

Medical School:	Chicago Medical School, Univ. of Health Sciences
Residency:	Boston University Affiliated Hospitals, Boston MA
	Fellowship: Shriner's Burn Institute, Boston, MA
Certified:	American Board of Plastic Surgery
Excels in:	Liposuction, Abdominoplasty, Facelift, Blepharoplasty, Breast Augmentation/reduction

Dr. Stevens has always been one of the surgeons I refer my liposuction clients to. He is the Master of the Cannula. I have no worry or concern that the suction cannula will be thrust only in areas of fat, not blood vessel or organ.

Dr. Gary Tearston
436 N. Bedford Dr. Ste. 203
Beverly Hills, CA 90210
310 659 5502

Secondary education:	Univ. of Southern California B.A. Economics
Medical School:	University of Pennsylvania Dr. of Medicine
Internship:	L.A. County Univ. of So. CA Chief Resident
Residency:	L.A. County Univ. of So. CA
Certifications:	Diplomate American Board Of General Surgery Diplomate American Bd. Of Plastic Surgery Diplomate National Board of Medical Examiners.
Honoria:	Chief of Plastic Surgery Div. Cedars-Sinai Med. Center 1998-2001
Excels at:	Facelift, Rhinoplasty, Breast Reconstruction, Lip Lift, Blepharoplasty

Dr. Tearston has been a beacon of plastic surgery in Beverly Hills for over 40 years. His expertise is well documented for procedures of the entire body. He enjoys his work, delights in making women beautiful, and has a warm, charming personality.

I provided aftercare to Dr. Tearston's patients for 18 years and always found him to be totally involved with his patient's surgical experience from pre-op to full recovery. You will have the utmost in confidence that you are in skilled, caring hands.

Dr. Robin T. W. Yuan
462 N. Linden Dr. Ste. 236
Beverly Hills, CA 90212
310 385 8425

Medical School:	Harvard College AB Biology
	Harvard Medical School 1978
	Post Doctoral Training UCLA
General Surgery Res.:	Cedars Sinai Medical Center
Plastic Surgery Res.:	Jackson Memorial Hosp., Miami, FL
Member:	American Society of Plastic Surgeons
	American Board of Facial, Plastic and
	Reconstructive Surgery
Excels at:	Breast Augmentation, Coronal,
	Mastopexy, Liposuction, Thigh
	Lift, Facelift, Abdominoplasty,
	Otoplasty, Rhinoplasty

Dr. Yuan is a committed, professional plastic surgeon. Each patient, each procedure, is of utmost importance to him. His skill as a surgeon is unquestionable. He is attentive, has a gentle demeanor invoking confidence and trust. He is exceptionally adept at surgery of the face.

7. *What are the potential complications and will you predetermine that I am a good medical candidate?*

8. *Where will the surgery be performed and who will be in attendance? If it is in a hospital then call that hospital and verify if the surgeon has privileges to perform the specific procedure.*

9. *When and how many times will he see you post-operatively?*

10. *What will my recovery period entail: pain/swelling/degree of discomfort/time lost from society/when can I go back to work?*

11. *Be critical of surgeons who promote liposuction as a method of major weight loss.*

Remember, more than likely you are paying for this consultation. Do not be embarrassed to ask the above pertinent questions. The surgeon understands that this is elective surgery and you are at will to select the surgeon of your choice. It is normal for him to want your patronage, but he is also aware that it is advantageous to be truthful and ethical at this time or it will only come back to haunt him should he not. Qualified surgeons have no reason to misrepresent.

Even legitimately qualified surgeons can have patients who develop complications. Be cautious of any surgeon who "guarantees" results, no matter what his certifications are.

As with any surgical procedures, complications are a consideration. Make sure you are in good medical health and your surgeon has taken the necessary lab tests to verify blood analysis and cardiac function. Be totally honest when discussing your medical history with him/her. Infections are also a consideration. Follow your surgeon's instructions, take your medications, and perform all treatments ordered. Make arrangements for your first post-operative night, do not "go it alone". Do not risk your results by fainting, resulting in damage to the surgical site or additional bodily harm. This book was written to amuse and educate you on the pleasures, pain, benefits, and risks of thwarting Grandmother Nature.

Glossary Of Terms

Abdominoplasty	Tummy tuck
Blepharoplasty	Eyelid Surgery
Breast Augmentation	Breast Implants
Coronal	Forehead lift with removal of scalp wedge
Endoscopic Forehead	Raising the forehead with the use of an endoscope and screws
Liposuction	SAL Suction Assisted Lipectomy, suctioning out of fat
Malarplasty	Cheek Implants
Mastopexy	Breast Lift
Meloplasty	Facelift
Mentoplasty	Chin Augmentation, implant
Otoplasty	Pinning back the ears
Phenol Peel	Deep chemical peel

Reduction Mammoplasty	Breast Reduction
Rhinoplasty	Nose Surgery
Rhytidectomy	Facelift
Submentoplasty	Sculpting of the neck
TCA Peel	Trychloracetate, light peel

About the Author

Maggie Lockridge, R.N., administered to the needs of the cosmetic surgical patient for eighteen years. She graduated as a Registered Nurse from St. Elizabeth's Hospital in Boston, MA, was an Industrial Nurse at the General Motors Futurama Pavilion during the World's Fair in Flushing N.Y., and worked in the operating room of Sloan Memorial Cancer Research Hospital in N.Y.C. She joined the U.S.A.F.N.C. and married a fighter pilot in 1967. They were blessed with two beautiful children and raised them in Hawaii.

Maggie moved to Los Angeles and spent the next seven years as Charge Nurse and then Administrator of Le Petit Ermitage, what was then Beverly Hills leading cosmetic surgery recovery retreat, located in the exclusive L'Ermitage Hotel.

When Le Petit closed it's doors and Maggie opened Chantique in 1994, she put together a warm and nurturing staff to tend to her guests' every need. Chantique offered its services to the patients of more than sixty cosmetic surgeons. Maggie oversaw the needs of guests from around the country and from every corner of the world. Some of Maggie's Beverly

Hill's guests stayed with her every 3-5 years over the eighteen years and she was referred to by writers as "The most recognized and least acknowledged woman in Beverly Hills." Thousands of women of Beverly Hills had been her guests and under her care, but no one acknowledged her in public as everyone's beauty was "God given". Maggie respected their privacy.

Her guest list ranged from actors and actresses, business men and women, politicians, the socially prominent and to men and women from all walks of life who desired to fight Grandmother Nature or embellish her work. Los Angeles has been designated as the cosmetic surgery capital of the world with more surgical procedures taking place there than any other city. Maggie feels that her job was unique to her profession and could probably only succeed in the city of beauty, Los Angeles.

www.ingramcontent.com/pod-product-compliance
Lightning Source LLC
Chambersburg PA
CBHW032010170526
45157CB00002B/635